DATE DUE

GREEN GORILLA

D1466662

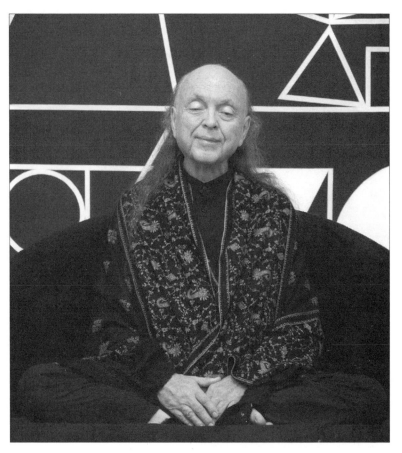

His Divine Presence
The Divine Avataric World-Teacher
RUCHIRA AVATAR ADI DA SAMRAJ
Adi Da Samrajashram, 2008

GREEN GORILLA

The Searchless Raw Diet

Given By
His Divine Presence
The Divine Avataric World-Teacher
Ruchira Avatar Adi Da Samraj

THE DAWN HORSE PRESS
MIDDLETOWN, CALIFORNIA

NOTE TO THE READER

All who study the "Radical" Reality-Way of Adidam Ruchiradam or take up its practice should remember that they are responding to a Call to become responsible for themselves. They should understand that they, not Avatar Adi Da Samraj or others, are responsible for any decision they make or action they take in the course of their lives of study or practice.

The devotional, Spiritual, functional, practical, relational, and cultural practices and disciplines referred to in this book are appropriate and natural practices that are voluntarily and progressively adopted by members of the practicing congregations of Adidam (as appropriate to the personal circumstance of each individual). Although anyone may find these practices useful and beneficial, they are not presented as advice or recommendations to the general reader or to anyone who is not a member of one of the practicing congregations of Adidam. And nothing in this book is intended as a diagnosis, prescription, or recommended treatment or cure for any specific "problem", whether medical, emotional, psychological, social, or Spiritual. One should apply a particular program of treatment, prevention, cure, or general health only in consultation with a licensed physician or other qualified professional.

Green Gorilla is formally authorized for publication by the Ruchira Sannyasin Order of Adidam Ruchiradam. (The Ruchira Sannyasin Order of Adidam Ruchiradam is the senior Cultural Authority within the formal gathering of formally acknowledged devotees of His Divine Presence, the Divine Avataric World-Teacher, Ruchira Avatar Adi Da Samraj.)

Produced by the Dawn Horse Press,
a division of the Avataric Pan-Communion of Adidam.

International Standard Book Number: 978-1-57097-256-0
Library of Congress Control Number: 2008931930

CONTENTS

ABOUT THE COVER

W*hat do gorillas eat? What are the primates who are close to the human form doing? They are practicing a raw diet. They haven't a clue about how to build a fire and cook something. They move about, so that they are constantly foraging in different places and taking food from different sources. The gorilla's diet is dominantly greens. Secondarily, the diet of the gorilla makes use of various kinds of fruits and seeds....The raw diet is something like an in-the-wild diet.*

—Ruchira Avatar Adi Da Samraj

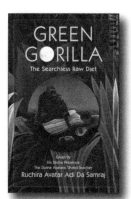

The image of a peaceful gorilla has been a theme of Avatar Adi Da's Instruction about diet since the late 1970s. His first published book about diet was entitled *The Eating Gorilla Comes In Peace*, followed several years later by the smaller *Raw Gorilla*. The present volume gives His further and most recent Instruction, emphasizing the simple and "searchless" approach to diet, as well as the importance of green leafy vegetables in the searchless raw dietary approach.

The inset image on the cover of this book is based on Henri Rousseau's painting *The Sleeping Gypsy*—with a peaceful gorilla in place of Rousseau's lion. This inset also directly ties *Green Gorilla* to the larger text *The Eating Gorilla Comes In Peace*—Avatar Adi Da's full address to "radical" health practice, including right diet. ∎

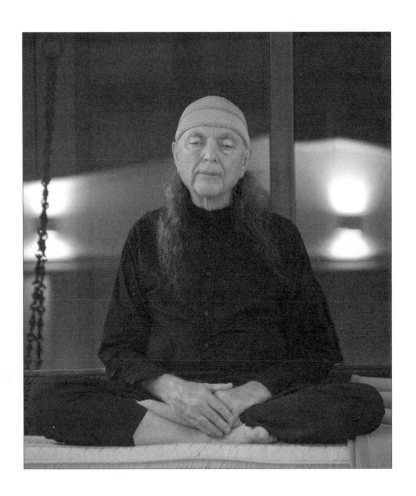

INTRODUCTION

by Daniel Bouwmeester, MD

The Discourses in this book were freely spoken by His Divine Presence Ruchira Avatar Adi Da Samraj in March and April of 2008, in a setting most appropriate to their theme. In a secluded stretch of Adi Da Samrajashram (the Fijian Island of Naitauba), Avatar Adi Da has established a forest hermitage known as "Lion's Lap". This beautiful environment is embraced by the canopy of green branches and leaves of the ancient, great trees overhead, and grasses and multi-colored flowers blanket the ground. In this pristine domain, the deep, silent Radiance of Avatar Adi Da's Blessing and Divine State is profoundly felt, Pervading everything and yet Prior to the body and the mind. It was in this circumstance that Avatar Adi Da was spontaneously moved to speak of lawful accord with the "green domain".

Avatar Adi Da has long been an advocate of the raw diet (a diet based on the principle of eating foods only in their "raw", or uncooked, state). Avatar Adi Da first communicated about the searchless approach to diet in *The Eating Gorilla Comes In Peace* (first printed in 1979) and He fully outlined and elaborated a raw dietary approach in *Raw Gorilla* (first printed in 1982). He has consistently communicated that, after an appropriate period of adaptation, the raw diet is the right and lawful diet for humankind.

Because of the Prior Nature of His Divine Condition, Avatar Adi Da is thoroughly experienced with what works for the body in its conformity and service to the Living Reality. Furthermore, He is sensitive to and eloquently critical of all the pitfalls, misinformation, hype, and seeking communicated everywhere, including in the "movement" associated with raw food.

Since the publication of *Raw Gorilla* in the early 1980s, the raw food movement has grown from being a "fringe" dietary approach (generally unknown or at best suspicious) to becoming more acceptable—almost mainstream. Raw food restaurants are now common in many cities. Raw food advocates are positively received on TV talk shows or in the media—and their presentations and books are easily found on the Internet. Some celebrities will not travel without their raw food chef!

Raw food advocates, in their attempt to be heard, have amassed a large body of scientific and empirical support for the validity of the raw food dietary approach. Many books and websites intelligently outline the scientific and practical basis for the raw diet and give testimonials not only for the usefulness of raw diet in helping to correct health conditions but also as a way to maintain optimum health and vitality. Old fears (of becoming emaciated or osteoporotic) and misinformation about the raw diet (such as the diet being deficient in protein and vitamin B12) have been addressed, encouraging many to make the transition to a totally or maximally raw diet.

Of course, concurrent with the growing number of public advocates of the raw diet is an ever-increasing number of different (and sometimes conflicting or confusing) approaches to the raw diet—some championing individual preference (or even the "instinctive" use of smell and taste) to select foods; some countering with prescribed proportions of fruits, vegetables, and oils; some suggesting various grasses, or sprouts, or blended drinks, as essential to the sustainability of the diet; and so on. One approach to popularizing the raw diet has been preparing raw foods in an increasingly gourmet manner. In His consideration of the raw diet—in this book and in His Teaching altogether—Avatar Adi Da addresses each of these approaches and more.

The common reasons promoted for embracing the raw diet are full of "promise"—raw diet is sometimes even approached as a religion in and of itself. Typically, raw diet is suggested for those who want to get healthy. Or it is argued that raw diet best supports unity with nature. Raw diet advocates sometimes suggest that the diet increases sensitivity to the breath and its influence on the body and personal energy. Some say that the raw diet supports or causes a deepening sensitivity to the "spirit", or heightens religious impulses. Some might even claim that raw food has something directly to do with enlightenment or truth.

At the same time that the raw food movement has been evolving, other common approaches to diet have also changed. Over the past thirty years, the medical profession has gone from being in "diet denial"—relative to the effect of diet on disease conditions—to emphasizing life-style changes for all the common chronic health problems. Accordingly, the standard conventional diets that are recommended by doctors have changed, now including many variations within the accepted standard (including diets like Atkins, South Beach, Pritikin, Metabolic, Blood Type, Zone, etc.). Another recommendation gaining ground is vegetarian (or plant-based) diet—also with many variations, including approaches that include dairy or eggs, the macrobiotic diet, the vegan diet, and numerous others.

Such a collage of dietary applications and seeking are but a narrow slice of the full spectrum of human pursuits that Avatar Adi Da Samraj has addressed in His years of Teaching-Work, beginning in 1972. Avatar Adi Da Submitted Himself to Teach those who—encumbered with all kinds of these common inclinations and established habit-patterns—came to Him for His evident Wisdom and Blessing. Over the years, as His Teaching-Submission continued, Avatar Adi Da fully addressed all matters that were brought to Him (including the matter of diet) to the point where His Teaching became summary—meaning that His Teaching had become clearly and finally established and He was no longer required to address points of view that were alternatives to His communicated and proven Way.

Avatar Adi Da's fundamental recommendation relative to diet is *the searchless raw (fructo-vegetarian) diet*—searchless in the sense that it is simply lawful management of a body in Communion with the Living Reality, free of the need to use food as a means to solve any kind of problem or seek any kind of ideal in body or mind. *Green Gorilla* is the essential, summary communication of the Divine Adept, Avatar Adi Da Samraj—to His devotees and to all—relative to diet.*

For those who are interested in a lawful, healthy life, there is great Wisdom here to guide you, free of any kind of exaggerated seeking approach. For Avatar Adi Da's devotees, practicing the Reality-Realizing Way of Adidam Ruchiradam, the dietary discipline given here is embraced as part of an entire life of devotional conformity to Avatar Adi Da. Such "whole bodily" devotion—or responsive devotional obedience—is the natural and inherent movement of the devotee who recognizes the Divine Master as the Living and Prior Reality. In this disposition of recognition, the devotee is drawn beyond the ordinary impulses of body and mind, into the profound process of Transcendental Spiritual Blessing and Awakening that is the greatest Gift Avatar Adi Da Samraj is here to Give.

Listen carefully to Avatar Adi Da's precise Words of Instruction. Conform to His Help. Let His Criticism penetrate all old habits, dietary patterns, and ongoing bodily addictions. Allow diet to be the benign simplicity that it rightfully is—and let it serve the body's submission to What Is Prior and Beyond. ■

* The new edition of *The Eating Gorilla Comes In Peace*, forthcoming, expands on the approach to diet presented here and also presents Avatar Adi Da's Instructions relative to health altogether.

Daniel Bouwmeester, MD, received his medical degree from the University of Melbourne, Australia, in 1975. He became a devotee of Ruchira Avatar Adi Da in 1974, and after his residency moved to the United States to be closer to Avatar Adi Da and His gathering of devotees in California. Daniel was part of a small group that directly participated with Avatar Adi Da Samraj throughout His years of Teaching-Submission. Daniel currently serves in the Radiant Life Clinic, in Fiji and California, practicing medicine on the basis of Avatar Adi Da's "radical" approach to healing, and continues to be one of Avatar Adi Da's personal physicians.

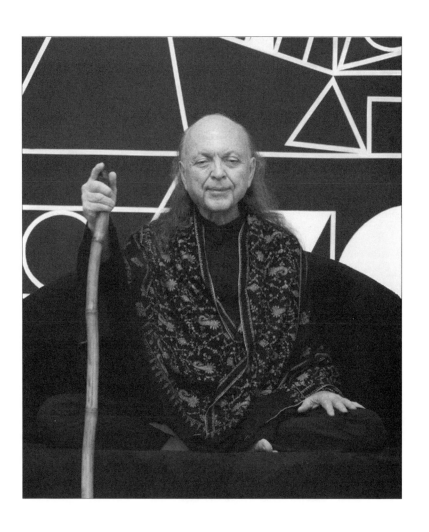

About His Divine Presence
Ruchira Avatar Adi Da Samraj
and the Reality-Way of Adidam Ruchiradam

*The Position of Reality Itself Is the Position of and
As That Which Is Always Already The Case....*

Reality Itself Is the Context of all "experiencing".

Reality Itself Is Truth.

*Reality Itself Is What is to be Realized—not merely
eventually, but always immediately, directly, and
tacitly.*

*That Reality Itself Is Truth Is the Realization
Sitting before you, in My Own Person.*

*The Divine Reality-Way of Adidam is Self-Revealed,
in Person, before your eyes.*

—His Divine Presence
Ruchira Avatar Adi Da Samraj
The Aletheon

Thousands of people have discovered the Truth for Real
when they encountered the Reality-Teaching of His
Divine Presence Ruchira Avatar Adi Da Samraj. And
Truth Itself is the Gift that Avatar Adi Da Samraj is here to
Offer to you.

Avatar Adi Da's entire Life—starting with His Illumined
birth on Long Island, New York, in 1939—has been devoted
to Communicating the Truth to others. He now Offers His
full Communication of Truth in the many books of His
Reality-Teaching. Taken together, His books offer His complete Revelation of the Way He Offers to all—the "Radical"
Reality-Way of Adidam Ruchiradam.

All of Avatar Adi Da's Words are an invitation to consider the Truth of Reality. And, even more than that, all of Avatar Adi Da's Words are an invitation to enter into a real and profound Spiritual relationship with Him—for He has always said, "I Offer you a relationship, not a technique."

Many who have started by reading Avatar Adi Da's Words have gone on to enter into this relationship as His formal devotees, practicing the Reality-Way of Adidam. And they have done so because they made the most profound discovery of their lives:

Avatar Adi Da Samraj is not merely a highly developed human being. He is able to speak the Truth for Real because He Is Himself the Living Divine Truth, Appearing on Earth in human form. In other words, He Is Reality Itself, the Very Truth of Existence—Appearing bodily for a time in our midst, in order to Reveal to all the Way to Realize Perfect Freedom.

Avatar Adi Da Samraj does not ask you to merely believe this about Him. Rather, He invites you to enter the Sphere of His Blessing—by freely considering His Words, and fully feeling their impact on your life and your heart. ■

.

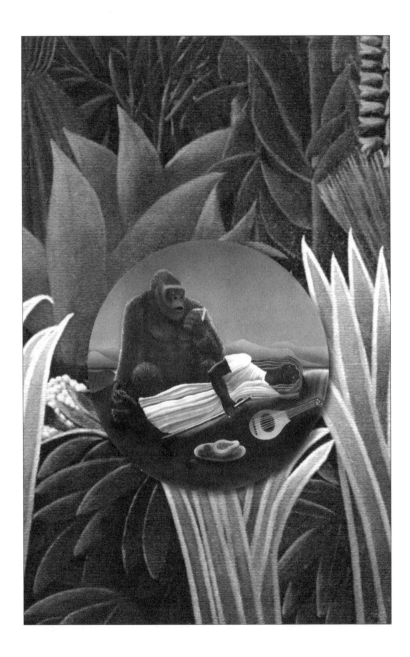

PART ONE

Principles of
the Searchless Raw Diet

The Right and Optimum Diet

From "The ego-'I' Is The Illusion of Relatedness"
by His Divine Presence
Ruchira Avatar Adi Da Samraj

The following essay is Ruchira Avatar Adi Da's summary Teaching on right diet, which lays the foundation for the rest of the Instruction and practical information in this book. In this essay, He speaks of the formal dietary discipline He Gives to His devotees in all four congregations of Adidam, which is also the diet He recommends for all human beings if they choose to consider and apply it. Avatar Adi Da says:

My "right life" Teachings apply to everyone. People do not necessarily have to become My devotees at the moment to benefit from these Teachings. Right life is not only something for My devotees to do—it is something for everyone to do. It applies to My devotees in their right-life obedience to Me because it is, in principle, right life. And if My Instruction is, in principle, right life, then anybody can do it.

—His Divine Presence
Ruchira Avatar Adi Da Samraj
June 1, 2008

Note also that the editors have added subheadings with key points to highlight the various topics within this essay.

The Gross Body Is the Food-Body

• The physical body is made of and depends on food.

• The quality of food eaten basically determines the state of the body, emotions, and thoughts.

• The "food-principle" is the fundamental basis for all physical healing.

The grossest dimension of the body-mind-complex is the physical body itself. It is associated with desire (or motive) and action based on desire. Therefore, the traditional path called "Karma Yoga" (or renunciation of the purposes and goals of the ego in the midst of bodily activity)* was developed as a means to transcend bondage to bodily desire and activity (by surrendering the "causes" and the "results" of bodily action to the Divine—and this by converting all actions into forms of worship). Similarly, in the only-by-Me Revealed and Given "Radical" Reality-Way of Adidam, My devotee converts all of his or her actions into forms of (ego-surrendering, ego-forgetting, and ego-transcending) "radical" (or always "at-the-root") devotion to Me.

The gross body is, very simply, the food-body. The gross body (itself) depends on (and is made of) food. The quality and quantity of food largely (or very basically) determines the state and desire and action of the physical body and the sense-mind. If food-taking is intelligently minimized, and if the food selected is both pure and purifying, then the physical

---

* The Hindu tradition speaks of four principal Spiritual paths (or four principal aspects of the Spiritual path). Karma Yoga is literally the "Yoga of action", in which every activity, no matter how humble, is transformed into ego-transcending service to the Divine. (The other three paths are Bhakti Yoga, the path of devotion, Raja Yoga, the path of higher psychic discipline, and Jnana Yoga, the path of transcendental insight.)

body (and, therefore, also the brain), and, thus and thereby, the entirety of the body-brain-based patterning of emotion and mind, passes through a spontaneous natural cycle that shows (progressive) signs of (first) purification, (then) rebalancing, and (finally) rejuvenation. Therefore, if food-taking is controlled, the body-mind-complex itself (including its thoughts, its desires, and even all of its activities) becomes directly (and, thus, at least in principle, rather easily) controllable—because it is, in fact, controllable, and (altogether) controllable by direct (and, thus, simple) means.

Because of this direct relationship between food-taking and the physical body, it is (in principle) very simple to restore the gross body to balance, health, and well-being. The basic treatment of any unhealthful condition of the gross body is a food-treatment (generally accompanied by rest from—or, otherwise, right and effective control of—all the enervating influences and effects of daily life). Therefore, primarily, it is through the food-discipline (accompanied by general "self"-discipline) that gross bodily purification, rebalancing, and rejuvenation are accomplished.

This "food-principle" is the fundamental physical basis of all physical healing. Some bodily conditions may require special healing treatments, but even such special approaches will be useful (in the fullest and long-term sense) only if accompanied by fundamental changes in diet (and simultaneous changes in one's habits of life). Therefore, always, the primary (and right) approach to physical health and physical well-being must be (first) to address (or examine) and (then) to treat (and to discipline) the gross body simply (or directly) as a food-process.

The Dimensions of the Body-Mind-Complex

Avatar Adi Da describes three fundamental dimensions of experience:

1. **gross**
2. **subtle**
3. **causal**

The **gross** (or outer) dimension corresponds to the physical level of experience and the waking state.

The **subtle** (or inner) dimension includes the dimension of life-energy and emotion and also everything to do with mind—both the conceptual mind and the domain of dreaming and psychic experience, including the range of supernormal experience that is commonly called "mystical".

The **causal** (or root) dimension refers to the depth where the "root" (or "causative") act of attention occurs in Consciousness—giving rise to the sense of the dichotomy between "I" and "other". This original (and always constant) act of separation is the "root"-form of the contraction as a separate self, and (therefore) the "root" of human suffering.

No level of the human structure is, in and of itself, Spiritual or Divine. Thus, none of the body-mind structures are the means or method of transformation in the Reality-Way of Adidam that is Given by Avatar Adi Da Samraj. Rather, the entire being is devotionally turned (and, thereby, surrendered) to Avatar Adi Da. His Transcendental Spiritual Blessing is the "Bright" Itself, Beyond all the structures of the "self"-contracted body-mind—gross, subtle, and causal.

The life-disciplines of Adidam—including the searchless raw diet—are a means of turning the faculties of the body-mind to Avatar Adi Da, particularly in the context of the gross dimension (or "gross body"). ■

The Yoga of Right Diet

• Right diet is thus a physical means for conforming the body to the process of Realizing Reality Itself.

The Yoga of right diet is a principal physical means (in the only-by-Me Revealed and Given Reality-Way of Adidam) whereby the body is utterly conformed to the Purpose of Most Perfect Realization of Reality Itself, Which Is Truth Itself, or Real (Acausal) God. The ego would adapt the body-mind-complex to purposes of "worldly" fulfillment and mere survival, but My devotee who rightly, truly, fully, and fully devotionally resorts to Me (and who, thus and thereby, understands egoity) no longer limits the body-mind-complex to merely conventional and "worldly" purposes, but (rather) makes the body into a Transcendentally-Spiritually-Activated and fully Yogically responsible body, through the exercise of "radical" devotion to Me (supported by all the disciplines of "conductivity" practice).*

Among all the functional, practical, relational, and cultural disciplines that serve the practice of the only-by-Me Revealed and Given Reality-Way of Adidam, the conservative discipline (or control) of diet is (elementally) the most basic—because dietary practice (which controls, or largely determines, the state of the food-body, or the state and general activity of the physical body) also determines the relative controllability of social, sexual, emotional, mental, and all other functional desires and activities.

If diet is controlled, the gross food-body is more easily controlled, and all the disciplines of the body-mind-"self" will be (to that degree) quickened in their effectiveness.

* See glossary for definitions of the practices of "radical" devotion to Avatar Adi Da as well as "conductivity" practice.

Therefore, in the only-by-Me Revealed and Given Reality-Way of Adidam, right and optimum dietary discipline is a necessary basic aspect of practice. . . .

Right Diet Does Not Burden the Body

• Right diet is conservative; purifying, rebalancing, and rejuvenating; and, in traditional language, "sattvic".

The right and optimum diet is (necessarily) a conservative diet. In right (or effective) practice of the Reality-Way of Adidam, dietary discipline fully serves the submission of personal energy and attention to the great process that becomes (Ultimately, by Means of My Divine Avataric Transcendental Spiritual Grace) Most Perfect Divine Self-Realization. Therefore, in the only-by-Me Revealed and Given Reality-Way of Adidam, the right and optimum diet must be intelligently moderated in its quantity and carefully selected in its quality, so that it will not burden the physical body or bind the mind (or attention) through food-desire and negative (or constipating, toxifying, and enervating) food-effects (and ingestion-effects in general), and so that (along with the necessary additional "consideration" and really effective transcending of addicted, aberrated, anxious, or even excessively private habits and patterns relative to food-taking and waste-elimination) it serves the yielding (or freeing) of functional human energy and attention to the Great (and, necessarily, devotionally Me-recognizing and devotionally to-Me-responding) Process of the intrinsic and fully life-effective transcending of the ego-"I". Consequently, right and optimum diet must be pure and purifying, rebalancing, and rejuvenating—and, therefore, natural, fresh, whole, wholesome, balanced, balancing, and non-toxic—or, in the language of the Asian Indian tradition, "sattvic".* And right and optimum diet must be limited to what is necessary and sufficient for bodily (and general psycho-physical) purification, balance, well-being, and appropriate service.

Eat Only Raw Foods

• The basic dietary orientation recommended by Avatar Adi Da Samraj is to eat only raw foods—principally vegetables (especially greens) and fruits.

• Food is taken in moderate amounts.

• Vitamins and supplements are only used if rightly medically advised.

• If a caffeine stimulant is required for functional or medical reasons, white or green (or possibly pu-erh) tea should be used (not coffee or black or oolong tea).

In the only-by-Me Revealed and Given Reality-Way of Adidam, the discipline of right ("minimum optimum") diet requires conformation to My herein-Given general dietary Instructions, in order to serve (in every present moment) the necessities of maximum good health, maximum well-being, and right full practice of the Reality-Way of Adidam, in the case of the individual. Thus, in the Reality-Way of Adidam, there is a basic dietary orientation (to which each individual must always directly adapt), and that basic orientation is Given by Me as a dietary rule and guide for all formally acknowledged practitioners of the Reality-Way of Adidam. That basic orientation (or dietary rule) is to eat only raw (and,

---

* "Sattvic" is an adjectival form of the Sanskrit noun "sattva". In the Hindu tradition, "sattva" is the principle of equilibrium (or harmony), one of the three qualities (or "gunas") of conditionally manifested existence—together with inertia (or "tamas") and activity (or "rajas").

altogether, pure and purifying) foods, consisting principally of vegetables (and, in particular, greens) and fruits, together with seeds and (in moderate quantities) nuts.

In the only-by-Me Revealed and Given Reality-Way of Adidam, the basic diet . . . is (in the general case) the diet that most fully and consistently meets all the requirements for right diet (or the "minimum optimum", and, as a general daily rule, consistently pure and purifying, rebalancing, and rejuvenative diet) I herein Indicate. That diet (the healthful virtues of which have been fully "experientially" Confirmed by Me, as well as by tradition, and by "modern" research and experimentation) is the raw fructo-vegetarian diet—consisting totally of raw (or uncooked, or unfired, and, thus, entirely living) foods. That basic (or "minimum optimum") diet consists principally of greens and fruits, together with seeds, nuts, sprouts, grasses, and other vegetables.* In the case of this by-Me-Given dietary discipline, foods are taken in solid or liquid or blended forms (except during fasts, or during any period in which an exclusively juiced liquid fruit, or liquid vegetable, or liquid fruit-and-vegetable diet is preferred), and food is always to be taken only in moderate amounts, using vitamins or other supplements only if (rightly) medically so advised. (On the relatively rare occasions when a caffeine-containing psycho-physical stimulant is rightly and truly required, for either functional or medicinal reasons, either green tea, or white tea, or, more rarely, pu-erh tea—all of which are generally regarded to have relatively non-toxic properties—may be taken. Because of their rather aggressively toxic properties, neither black tea nor oolong tea nor coffee should, as a general rule, be taken.)

---

* To the maximum extent possible, all raw living foods should be locally grown (or, if imported, not adulterated in travel), pesticide-free, grown in a sustainable manner, not genetically modified or irradiated, and entirely non-toxic.

Blended Green Drinks

• Prepare blended green drinks with (principally) greens, fruit to taste, and pure water. (Variations and other additions are described in the text.)

• Drink approximately 1 to 2 quarts (or 1 to 2 liters) of green drink per day.

A principal element of the raw fructo-vegetarian dietary practice I have Given is the regular (daily) use of "blended green drinks", made (most commonly) of green leafy vegetables and sweet fruits.* "Green drinks" provide a highly concentrated form of the nutrients found in green leafy vegetables—generally in much greater quantity than could be ingested by eating the greens whole. The sweet fruits are added to "green drinks" in order to make the concentrated greens palatable, and also to provide additional nutrients and calories.

Blended "green drinks" are prepared using one or more varieties of green leafy vegetables—using whatever edible greens are available.† In temperate climates, appropriate edible greens include such plants as kale, chard, spinach, lettuce, collard greens, bok choy, and so on. Edible weeds (including, in temperate zones, such plants as dandelion, lambsquarters, plantain, and so on), herbs (such as dill, basil, cilantro, mint, parsley, and so on), sprouts (such as

---

* Note that "sweet fruits" is being used here as a generic term, and not as a specific technical term contrasting with "acid fruits", etc. Rather, it is contrasting with "non-sweet" or seeded vegetable-fruits.

† Again, it is important that such greens be, as much as possible, locally grown (or, if imported, not adulterated in travel), pesticide-free, grown in a sustainable manner, not genetically modified or irradiated, and entirely non-toxic.

alfalfa, clover, buckwheat, sunflower, and so on), other vegetables (such as celery, cucumber, and so on), and medicinal plants (such as aloe vera) may also be added to a "green drink".

It is important to rotate the type of greens used, in order to avoid any over-accumulation in the body of the different naturally-occurring alkaloids contained in each variety of greens. Such an imbalance may lead to a disinclination to eat a particular green (indicating that it should be avoided for a time).*

In addition to the greens, one or more fruits (such as apple, pineapple, banana, papaya, mango, pear, lemon, berries, and so on) are to be added, to taste—together with sufficient pure water for blending the drink to the desired consistency.

It is important that the "green drink" be thoroughly blended, in order to optimize the assimilation of nutrients. The total daily intake of "green drinks" should be one to two quarts (32–64 oz., or 1–2 liters) or more, progressively consumed over a total of three or more occasions each day.

Further healthful additions to the basic "green drink" are also possible, such as a spoonful of ground flaxseed, chlorella, spirulina, or blue-green algae, a moderate amount of wheatgrass juice or lemon juice or lime juice, and so on. It is also possible to prepare blended "green drinks" without sweet fruits—and, in the case of individuals who have a bodily reaction to sweet fruits, this may be a necessary substitution—using, instead, seed-bearing vegetables (or "vegetable fruits", such as cucumbers, tomatoes, bell peppers, and so on) or other types of vegetables (such as celery).†

---

* See Victoria Boutenko's book *Green for Life* for more information on this point.

† Green drinks are described in more detail in part 3 of this book (see pp. 114–15) and in *The Eating Gorilla Comes In Peace* (forthcoming).

Balancing Fruit and Vegetable Meals

• Through alternating fruit and vegetable meals, find a balance of fruits and vegetables that works based on individual sensitivity.

In the raw fructo-vegetarian dietary practice I have Given, each meal should generally consist either of sweet fruits or of vegetables (including seed-bearing vegetables, or "vegetable fruits"). The choice of which type of meal to eat on any particular occasion or at any particular time of day, as well as which specific fruits or vegetables are optimal for the individual, is a matter that must be determined by sensitivity to the body's signs.

Fruit meals may consist either of a single fruit or of a variety of fruits—such as apples, pears, berries, cherries, bananas, tropical fruits, and so on. Fruit meals may also consist of melons or citrus fruits, either of which should generally be taken alone, for optimum digestibility.

Vegetable meals consist principally of seed-bearing vegetables (or "vegetable fruits", such as tomatoes, cucumbers, zucchini, bell peppers, and so on), together with lettuces and other greens—with smaller quantities of stem vegetables (such as celery or asparagus), and root vegetables (such as carrots, beets, and jicama). Vegetable meals should not include either tuberous (and excessively starchy) vegetables (such as potatoes and yams) or the pungent (and inter-brain-blocking*) bulb vegetables (such as onions, garlic, and leeks). "Vegetable fruits" may also be included in a fruit meal.

---

* Despite arguments in favor of the health properties of "pungent" vegetables, such as garlic, there is traditional recommendation against their "stimulating" properties in the context of authentic Spiritual practice. Also, modern research by individuals such as Robert (Bob) C. Beck, D.Sc. (1925–2002), indicates that pungent vegetables impede the communication between the two hemispheres of the brain.

Either type of meal may include sprouts and (in moderate quantity) seeds. Nuts are best combined with vegetable meals, or (otherwise) taken alone. As a general rule, fatty foods (including seeds, nuts, and avocados) would be minimized to approximately ten percent of daily caloric intake. (For most optimum absorption of nutrients and digestibility, seeds and nuts may be taken in soaked form.)

Through the alternation of fruit meals and vegetable meals (in the by-Me-Given raw fructo-vegetarian dietary practice), there should, in the case of most individuals, be a generally equal balance between sweet fruits and vegetables. Such is a basic, straightforward, and typical approach— although some individuals may find that it is optimal to adopt an almost exclusively fruitarian approach to meals (apart from the greens and other vegetables taken in "green drinks"). When the raw fructo-vegetarian diet is rightly applied, the body should be consistently energized, but not in a stressful manner. Thus, the feeling of energized well-being is the day to day measure by which the individual should choose between fruit meals and vegetable meals.

An imbalance of any particular type of food in the diet may have enervating or toxifying effects in the body. For example, an excess of sweet fruits can be overly purifying and create enervation in the body, whereas an excess of nuts or seeds can create signs of toxicity in the body. Therefore, it is important for each individual to balance the amounts of (primarily) fruits and greens, as well as (secondarily) seeds, nuts, and other vegetables, based on sensitivity to the body's signs from day to day—rather than attempt to hold to any absolute measure (or prescribed formula) of balance between the different types of raw foods.

Understand This Dietary Design

• Cooking food destroys enzymes, vitamins, and nutrients.

• Study Avatar Adi Da's Word on the searchless raw diet, and (with discrimination) the literature He has recommended about diet from others.

• Artfully establish the diet, accounting for the various factors of your environment and body type.

• Get right, professional medical supervision from individuals who are knowledgeable about Avatar Adi Da's dietary approach.

The basic rule of the (generally, consistently neither overeating nor undereating) "minimum optimum" dietary design is that food should be restricted to raw substances, generally limited to the range of possibilities I have Described.

The reason that the cooking, or firing, of foods is, in general, not optimal is that heat destroys the enzymes, heat-sensitive vitamins, and other heat-sensitive nutrients naturally present in raw foods, and it also changes the chemical structure of proteins and sugars in raw foods such that these proteins and sugars become less usable by—or, in some preparations, even harmful to—the body.*

---

* The effects cooking has on foods are discussed in such works as:

The Sunfood Diet Success System: 36 Lessons in Health Transformation, by David Wolfe (San Diego, Calif.: Sunfood Publishing, 7th ed., 2008).

Eating for Beauty: For Women and Men, by David Wolfe (San Diego, Calif.: Maul Brothers Publishing, 2003).

Conscious Eating, by Gabriel Cousens (Berkeley, Calif.: North Atlantic Books, 2000), pp. 563–64.

Health Secrets from Europe, by Paavo O. Airola (New York: Arco Publishing, 1980), pp. 48–50.

In order to understand and evaluate the "minimum optimum" (pure and purifying, rebalancing, rejuvenating, and, as a general rule, totally raw) dietary discipline (or disciplined dietary practice) given by Me for application by all practitioners formally embracing the Reality-Way of Adidam (and Recommended by Me for application by all of humankind), you should study the total dietary approach Communicated in My Summaries of Instruction relative to dietary discipline.* Likewise, as a further aid to your understanding and evaluation of the by-Me-Given "minimum optimum" dietary discipline, you should (by means of a systematic, guided study of the traditional and "modern" literature I have Collected and Described for this purpose†) become familiar with the total tradition, including rightly-oriented "modern" research and experimentation, relative to pure and purifying, rebalancing, and rejuvenating dietary discipline. Such study is a useful support to your embrace of the by-Me-Given "minimum optimum" dietary discipline. I Call you to always intensively engage the by-Me-Given dietary discipline—always artfully (and appropriately, or as necessary, and without abandoning the by-Me-Given "minimum optimum" dietary principles) taking into account such present-time factors as climate and season, the availability (and the quality) of locally grown food, the availability (and the quality) of food in general, the level of your physical (and mental, and emotional) purification, the state of your health in general, the degree and kind of your daily activity, and even all the factors associated with your age, your degree of vitality,

---

* This book, along with the larger text *The Eating Gorilla Comes In Peace* (new edition forthcoming), is Avatar Adi Da's summary communication on dietary discipline (and health). A relatively brief summary of Avatar Adi Da's dietary Instruction is also found in Chapter 13 of *The Knee of Listening*.

† The "For Further Study" section of this book (pp. 130–34) includes a selection of such literature collected by Avatar Adi Da. The books on that list represent a variety of points of view and recommended approaches to diet. The inclusion of a title on that list does not mean that the views presented therein are "endorsed" by Avatar Adi Da Samraj, but (rather) that there is something about the contents of the book that is worth considering.

your psycho-physical type,* and your stage of practice-demonstration in the Reality-Way of Adidam.† And always practice the by-Me-Given dietary discipline with appropriate medical advice and supervision, so that the pace, the special requirements, and the results of your application of the by-Me-Given "minimum optimum" dietary discipline can be determined most efficiently and organized most effectively.

The Progress of Adaptation and Fasting

• First transition to the fructo-vegetarian diet that includes both cooked and raw foods, and from there to the totally raw food discipline.

• Use periodic fasting as an aid to the process of purification, rebalancing, and rejuvenation.

As a Second Congregation practitioner in the Reality-Way of Adidam (or as any individual who is applying himself or herself to this dietary discipline), begin (as a general rule) by adapting to and refining a basic fructo-vegetarian (fruit-and-vegetable) diet, which diet should (as a matter of initial adaptation) consist of both raw and cooked foods, and adapt to (and refine) that basic dietary practice as a progressively

---

* Avatar Adi Da has distinguished three basic psycho-physical types (or strategies), which He calls "vital", "peculiar", and "solid". The "vital" person is oriented to the physical dimension of existence, the "peculiar" person is oriented to the emotional dimension of existence, and the "solid" person is oriented to the mental dimension of existence. (For Avatar Adi Da's extended Instruction relative to these three psycho-physical types, see *The Dawn Horse Testament*.) While every individual is characteristically dominated by one of these three strategies, the three strategies are not mutually exclusive, and a combination of two or more strategies may need to be taken into account in modifying the diet.

† Avatar Adi Da describes how one's adaptation to the "minimum optimum" diet must be fully in place to transition to the First Congregation of the Reality-Way of Adidam. However, the "minimum optimum" diet is, by design, always purifying and rejuvenating, and, therefore, is constantly and progressively refined as one matures in the First Congregation process altogether.

all-raw dietary practice while you also adapt to and refine all the other basic and foundationary (functional, practical, relational, and cultural) requirements for "self"-discipline in the only-by-Me Revealed and Given Reality-Way of Adidam.*

Each and every practitioner of the only-by-Me Revealed and Given Reality-Way of Adidam is Called by Me (and is always to be formally expected) to constantly and intensively maintain the "self"-discipline of bodily purification, bodily rebalancing, and bodily rejuvenation (or bodily regeneration). As a basic means to quicken the effectiveness of your by-Me-Given (and formally expected) obligation to constantly and intensively maintain the "self"-discipline of bodily purification, bodily rebalancing, and bodily rejuvenation (or bodily regeneration), your dietary practice should also include right occasional and periodic fasting (unless you are otherwise rightly medically advised). Therefore, unless your bodily state (of <u>fully</u> achieved purification) and the purity of your daily food-intake do not (at any present moment) require it, your dietary practice should (in the general case) also (as necessary) include appropriate occasional (twenty-four-hour, or longer) and regular (extended) periodic fasting.† Long fasts are (in the general case) to be engaged periodically or at least once per year (unless right medical advice prohibits long fasts, or, otherwise, an exceptional state of bodily and dietary purity makes a long fast, in any present moment, unnecessary)—and, to be effective, long fasts should be continued for at least seven to ten days, and up to three or four weeks (or even longer). In addition,

---

* For a description of "all the other basic and foundationary . . . requirements for 'self'-discipline", please see *The Reality-Way of Adidam* (forthcoming 2008, The Dawn Horse Press).

† Such fasts should consist of the avoidance of all food intake—except for one or another (or, perhaps, a combination) of pure water, pure water with a small amount of lemon juice (or other citrus juice, or other fruit juice) added, pure water extracts of vegetables (otherwise known as "De la Torre" drinks), raw (and, perhaps, diluted) fruit juices, raw (and, perhaps, diluted) vegetable juices, and herb teas. See pp. 119–29 for more details on fasting.

shorter or longer periods of totally raw mono-diet* may also be engaged for the purpose of continuing the process of bodily purification during periods of time before and after fasting—but such temporary (rather than regular and constant) raw-mono-diet exercises should (in the general case) be engaged only <u>in addition</u> to fasting, and not as an <u>alternative</u> to fasting.

Refine (or simplify) your diet progressively, and, thus (but as directly and quickly as possible), pass through the necessary cycles of purification, rebalancing, and rejuvenation—until, in the course of Second Congregation practice of the Reality-Way of Adidam (or, otherwise, in the course of dietary adaptation engaged by any individual), the discipline of "minimum optimum" (and, as a general rule, <u>totally</u> raw) diet (in the manner that has been demonstrated to be right and appropriate in your particular case, including the appropriately alternated cycles of purification, rebalancing, and rejuvenation, and with food taken always in minimum, but adequate, quantities) is <u>stably</u> achieved. . . .

Justifiable Health Exceptions

• Adding cooked foods to the raw diet should be on the temporary basis of medical necessity, and the effects of using such foods should be carefully observed.

Any individual . . . who is medically (and <u>correctly</u>) advised to temporarily include a broader range of foods in his or her diet, as his or her right form (in the any given period of his or her life) of the "minimum optimum" approach to diet—including (perhaps) cooked foods, and (perhaps) milk and milk products, and (perhaps) also eggs,

---

* A purifying raw mono-diet is taking only a single kind of raw food for a period of time. See p. 129 for more details on mono-diet.

or (perhaps) even flesh food (whether fish, fowl, or animal), and (perhaps) with therapeutic doses of vitamins and other food supplements as well, in addition to a basic diet of greens, fruits, nuts, seeds, sprouts, and various other vegetables—may, of course, do so (under right medical supervision, and, in the case of My formally practicing devotees, as must be the case relative to even every matter of practice and discipline in the Reality-Way of Adidam, always with the formal agreement of the formal sacred cooperative cultural gathering of all formally acknowledged practitioners of the Reality-Way of Adidam), but they should do so without "self"-indulgence, and strictly for health reasons, and only as a temporary concession to necessity, and with constant sensitivity (and ego-transcending response) to the effects such foods produce in the body-mind-complex, and on personal energy, and on attention. In most cases, any such plan (if, rightly, medically required) would be related to the treatment either of some varieties of disease or of constitutional weakness that are (at least temporarily) not amenable to the all-raw (and, thus, optimally pure and purifying, rebalancing, and rejuvenative) dietary approach. . . .

Avoiding Use of Intoxicants and Drugs

• In the Reality-Way of Adidam, there is no use of intoxicants (with the rare possible exception of token amounts for sacred ceremonies), and absolutely no use of medically inappropriate drugs.

All formally acknowledged practitioners of the Reality-Way of Adidam must, as a consistent and absolute rule (established even from the beginning of each individual's formal acceptance into Second Congregation practice), entirely avoid (and are to be formally expected to, as a consistent and absolute rule, entirely avoid) all use (with the possible rare exception only of token and merely symbolic use, as may sometimes be required by custom for respectful and right participation in, necessarily rare, sacred, or entirely ceremonial and non-personal, social occasions) of the more common (or commonly used) intoxicants (such as tobacco, alcohol, or kava)—and this because the casual (and also cumulative) effects of these substances are deluding, degenerative, and unhealthful.

All formally acknowledged practitioners of the Reality-Way of Adidam must, as a consistent and absolute rule (established even from the beginning of an individual's formal acceptance into Second Congregation practice), entirely avoid (and are to be formally expected to, as a consistent and absolute rule, entirely avoid) all use of "soft" drugs (such as cannabis), all use of the traditional hallucinogenic drugs (such as peyote, mescaline, psilocybin, ayahuasca, and so on), all use of the hallucinogenic drugs that have a traditional social use in certain cultures (such as opium, and so on), all use of the so-called "recreational" (or even "hard") drugs (without any tradition of sacred or social use) that have been developed by means of chemical processes (such as heroin, cocaine, LSD, methamphetamines, and so on), all use of the so-called "recreational" (or even "hard") drugs originally developed for medical purposes (such as barbiturates and amphetamines), and (indeed) all use of any otherwise medically inappropriate drugs that may be discovered or developed at any point in human history—because the casual effects (and, in general, even the inherent characteristics) of "soft" drugs (such as cannabis), "recreational" drugs (of any kind), hallucinogenic drugs, "hard" drugs, and otherwise medically inappropriate drugs are (generally) extremely deluding, degenerative, and unhealthful.

Every practitioner formally embracing the Reality-Way of Adidam must always remember and actively (by right practice) affirm that the Reality-Way of Adidam is, even from the beginning, an intrinsically ego-transcending and (necessarily) psycho-physically purifying Way of life, based upon the Principle that Realization and Renunciation are (intrinsically and necessarily) the Same. Therefore, from the beginning of the Reality-Way of Adidam, the consistent avoidance of toxic (or otherwise gross and impure) substances is the necessary (and formally to be expected) rule of practice.

The Desensitizing Effects of Self-Indulgence

• Toxic substances (such as intoxicants and drugs) work against the effectiveness of practice of the Reality-Way of Adidam, by desensitizing the user of such substances to Avatar Adi Da— devotionally and Spiritually.

• The abandonment of toxic substances is not a matter of puritanical or moralistic body-denial, but rather of the homely and realistic and lawful discipline of the body-mind-complex.

My any devotee who persists in habits and addictions of gross physical "self"-indulgence (including dietary "self"-indulgence) is inevitably desensitized to Me—both devotionally and Transcendentally Spiritually. Therefore, such habits and addictions of gross physical "self"-indulgence undermine (and work against) the effectiveness of the Reality-Way of Divine Self-Realization That I have Given to My devotees. This is the reason why refinement of the physical body via a diet that is conservative (or "minimum optimum"), and (in the general case) fructo-vegetarian, and (in the general case) totally raw, and via a conservative (and truly pure and purifying) approach to food-taking (and body-maintenance altogether), is necessary in the only-by-Me Revealed and Given Reality-Way of Adidam.

Any use of even the more common (or commonly used) intoxicants (such as tobacco, alcohol, or kava), and (to an even greater degree) any use of "soft" drugs (such as cannabis), temporarily suppresses psycho-physical (and heart-specific, and brain-specific, and nervous-system-specific) sensitivity to My Divine Avataric Transcendental Spiritual Self-Transmission—after an initial period of gross intoxication, in which such sensitivity may, at the gross level, seem (to the temporarily intoxicated user) to increase. The perennial popular (or common) wisdom relative to the Law and Lesson of "fun" always applies. If you play—you must pay! If you dance—you must pay the piper! Even the executioner has his price! And the longer and hotter the dance, the more you must pay—whether now or later! And the longer you wait to pay your fees, the more the fees compound and increase!

Therefore (and not for any moralistic or puritanical or idealistic reasons), My devotee must establish toxin-free functional equanimity—thus and thereby allowing the magnification of true and full sensitivity to My Divine Avataric Transcendental Spiritual Self-Transmission, and the possibility of continuing and furthering the devotional and Transcendental Spiritual Process of Realizing Me.

The universal human (and ego-bound, and ego-binding) tendency to desensitize the body-mind-complex to Me through indulgence in gross (or degenerative) psycho-physical habits of any and every kind is the first and essential reason why (in the only-by-Me Revealed and Given Reality-Way of Adidam) there must be the right and consistent exercise of right and optimum disciplines of the gross physical (and of the entire body-mind-complex). Therefore, in the only-by-Me Revealed and Given Reality-Way of Adidam, the right and optimum disciplining of gross (or degenerative) psycho-physical habits in general, and of dietary "self"-indulgence in particular, is not a puritanical matter, or a moralistic matter—

nor is it an idealistic matter. My devotees are not Called by Me to discipline the body-mind-"self" as a form of psycho-physical negativity (or body-denial), or as a form of utopian search for perfection in the context of conditionally manifested existence. Rather, in the only-by-Me Revealed and Given Reality-Way of Adidam, the right and optimum disciplining of the body-mind-"self" (including the general, and right-principled, relinquishment of gross, or degenerative, psycho-physical habits, and the <u>consistent</u> whole bodily, or total psycho-physical, and altogether right-principled, embrace of truly right and optimum psycho-physical disciplines) is simply a necessary and homely part of the realistic, and practical, and really and practically ego-transcending approach to Me, and to the Real Process of devotional, and (in due course, as My Avatarically Self-Transmitted Divine Transcendental Spiritual Grace will Have It) Transcendental Spiritual, relationship to Me—which relationship (formally, and fully accountably, embraced and practiced), and not any mere "self"-applied and ego-serving (or ego-improving, or even body-mind-improving) "techniques", is (<u>itself</u>) the only-by-Me Revealed and Given Reality-Way of Adidam.

More About Adaptation to the Raw Diet

• The transition from a conventional diet to the searchless raw diet can take anywhere from several weeks to a couple of months or longer.

The total transition from conventional (or "worldly") dietary practice to practice of right "minimum optimum" (and, as a general rule, <u>totally</u> raw) diet is a matter of a properly planned (and, as necessary, even medically supervised) transitional process of functional (and even mental and emotional) adaptation. As a general rule, the course of dietary adaptation should readily and quickly proceed from basic fructo-vegetarian dietary practice to a totally raw fructo-vegetarian dietary practice (consisting principally of greens and fruits—with intensive daily use of "green drinks").

As a general rule, the process of adaptation to a fructo-vegetarian (fruit-and-vegetable) dietary practice that is consistently totally raw may rightly take from several weeks to between one and two months (or, in rare cases, even longer), with the actual transition-time determined by the previous habits, the strength of intention, and the general state of health of the individual. And, in <u>every</u> case, that practice-demonstration (or, otherwise, the right practice-demonstration of any medically necessary variation on the "minimum optimum" diet), when it is right and real and true, is always (and necessarily) associated with profound and life-practice-converting discoveries about the body-mind-"self"—such that further practice-demonstration in the Reality-Way of Adidam is (thereby) given an extraordinarily positively transformed psycho-physical basis.

"Lunch-Righteousness" Vs. Searchless Right Diet

- Avatar Adi Da's Instruction on diet is based on His own examination of all alternative approaches.

- His Instruction on diet is a Teaching-Message—about a searchless diet—not a message about "salvation through diet".

My Summary Instruction about the dietary discipline in the only-by-Me Revealed and Given "Radical" Reality-Way of Adidam is (like all the Instruction Given by Me relative to the functional, practical, relational, and cultural disciplines of the Reality-Way of Adidam) the result of many years of examining all potential alternative orientations—as part of My Own Divine Avataric Ordeal of Self-Awakened Adaptation and My Divine Avataric Self-Submission to Teach. Out of This Process came My Summary Communication about the principles of the "minimum optimum" (and totally raw) approach to dietary practice, as well as My Criticism of the dietary practice of the usual person, and even My Criticism of the false view (or misunderstanding) of diet as a so-called "Spiritual" practice.

I have used the term "lunch-righteousness" to describe the kind of mentality that seeks "salvation through diet". No seeking of any kind can be part of the Reality-Way of Adidam I have Revealed and Given. Rather, My Instruction on right and optimum diet is a Teaching-Message from Me— Given to My formally practicing devotees, and to all of humankind. Right and optimum diet is a form of searchless (and, thus, motiveless) right life. Right and optimum diet is a basic and inevitable part of the foundation practice of "self"-discipline in the only-by-Me Revealed and Given Reality-Way of Adidam, to be practiced by My devotee in devotional recognition-response to Me. My dietary Instruction is not, fundamentally, a message about health—although better health is certainly a characteristic result of the practice of such right diet. Rather, the by-Me-Given dietary discipline in the Reality-Way of Adidam is a devotional practice—and, therefore, it is a searchless and intrinsically ego-transcending practical discipline assumed on the basis of recognition-responsive whole bodily devotion to Me.

Exaggerated and Seeking Approaches to Diet

• Avatar Adi Da Calls for an understanding of various forms of seeking for health and well-being through diet.

• His Communication relative to diet is straightforward and not made "appealing" by "fascinating" means.

Right understanding and right practice of the dietary discipline in the only-by-Me Revealed and Given "Radical" Reality-Way of Adidam—and, indeed, right understanding and right practice of all forms of functional, practical, relational, and cultural "self"-discipline in the Reality-Way of Adidam—tends to be obscured by the search for health and personal well-being (or "self"-satisfaction). The lack of right understanding relative to practical "self"-discipline engenders all kinds of egoic misinterpretations relative to the right practice of "self"-discipline. Such is not the Reality-Way of Adidam That I have Revealed and Given, and My devotees must be sensitive to the tendency to abandon right understanding of the by-Me-Given forms of "self"-discipline. . . .

For instance, the discipline of right and optimum diet (generally speaking) is applied in the context of the first three stages of life, and, therefore, in the context of egoity in terms of the first three stages of life.* My Reality-Teaching about diet is, first of all, founded in devotion to Me, and, additionally, presents the principle of right and optimum diet through critical examination of the various egoic approaches to diet that characteristically arise in the context of the first three stages of life.

* In other words, dietary discipline is an address to the bodily, emotional, and mental aspects of the being in the waking state.

The Stages of Life

Avatar Adi Da Samraj has Revealed a precise "mapping" of the developmental possibilities of human experience in terms of six stages of life—which account for, and correspond to, all the dimensions of experience that are potential in the human structure. His own Divine Avataric Revelation—the Realization of the "Bright", Prior to all potential experience—is the seventh stage of life. Understanding this structure of seven stages illuminates the unique nature of the process of Adidam. For a complete description, see the glossary entry **stages of life**.

The first three (or foundation) stages of life constitute the ordinary course of human adaptation—characterized (respectively) by bodily, emotional, and mental growth. Each of the first three stages of life takes approximately seven years to be established. Every individual who lives to an adult age inevitably adapts (although, generally speaking, only partially) to the first three stages of life. In the general case, this is where the developmental potential stops—at the gross level of adaptation. Religions based fundamentally on beliefs and moral codes (without direct experience of the dimensions beyond the material world) belong to this foundation level of human development. ■

My Reality-Teaching about the necessary forms of "self"-discipline in the Reality-Way of Adidam is not merely a message about health. Obviously, My practical Instruction to My devotees relates to matters of health, but the improvement of one's health is not the principal purpose of the by-Me-Given forms of "self"-discipline. Likewise, My Divine Avataric Reality-Teaching cannot be reduced to an address to egoity merely in the mode of the first three stages of life, nor to an address to fantasies, illusions, or attachments relative to the patterns intrinsic to stages of life beyond the first three—nor is My Reality-Teaching to be made subordinate to messages coming from the existing "religious", Spiritual, and Transcendental traditions.

Much of the popular literature on diet that purports to relate to Spiritual practice—even much of the popular communications about vegetarian diet and raw diet altogether—tends to be associated with "lunch-righteousness", faddism, and hype, and even a kind of "messianic" approach to communicating about diet by people who are egoically deluded by their own energies.

My Communication about diet is not hyped. It is not offering "glorious salvation" by means of lunch. The bare facts of the dietary principles in the Reality-Way of Adidam are not, in and of themselves, particularly interesting, or made appealing by means of fascinating gimmicks. The principles of the right and optimum dietary approach I have Given are a very direct address to real matters of practical living—including, principally, many forms of My Criticism of egoity in the mode of "self"-indulgence and the misuse of diet as a form of consolation, as well as My Criticisms of faddism, or the search for "salvation through diet".

My Communication about diet is a straightforward approach that must be practiced with great intelligence and as part of a process of real "self"-observation, accountability within the cooperative cultural gathering of My devotees, and right medical guidance. My Communication about right and optimum diet is an Offering of specific principles that can be applied in every individual case.

Those who are vulnerable to fascination with diet and "lunch gurus" may tend to bring such notions to the study of My Instruction and try to find the same fascination in My Communications about right diet. Others, who are "self"-indulgent, resist the maintaining of "self"-discipline altogether. Both of these false approaches to dietary practice—the "messianic" (or "lunch-righteous") and the "self"-indulgent—are (and must be) Criticized by Me. Therefore, My Instruction relative to right diet addresses both tendencies toward exaggeration—either exaggeration via "self"-indulgence or exaggeration via the absurdity of "messianic lunchism" (or the illusion that diet somehow leads to Divine Self-Realization).

Right Diet Does Not "Cause" Realization

• Diet is a practical, biological matter—it is not causative in relation to the Transcendental Spiritual process of Realization itself.

Right diet does not (and cannot) "cause" Divine Self-Realization. In fact, right diet (in and of itself) has nothing to do with Divine Self-Realization (Itself). Therefore, in the only-by-Me Revealed and Given Reality-Way of Adidam, right diet is simply and only a practical discipline.

The principles of the practice of diet Communicated by Me are a basis for an intelligent approach to dietary practice. A characteristic of the dietary practice in the Reality-Way of Adidam is that it is without extremes. It is simply an intelligent approach to the matter. It is not a diet for seekers.

In making an intelligent approach to dietary practice, it is critically important that you rightly manage the transition from a conventional (or "worldly") diet to the raw fructo-vegetarian diet—otherwise, your unpreparedness will likely lead you to feel that the by-Me-Given dietary principles do not work in your case.

The raw fructo-vegetarian (and, altogether, "minimum optimum") dietary approach is part of My basic Instruction, and it is simply the form of dietary practice that naturally fits within the total structure of right principles I have Communicated.

Diet is a straightforward, practical matter—and the practice of right diet is likewise straightforward. One must learn about diet, of course, but the application of right dietary principles in practice should be so straightforward, from day to day, that the total life of right practice is not burdened with exaggerated attention to the physical dimension of the living being.

People who are intensely involved in dietary seeking are constantly occupied with their search. Such people become deluded by their own energies and fascinations, and they exaggerate the importance of diet—presuming, in fact, that diet has something to do with Spiritual Consciousness. Diet, in and of itself, has nothing to do with either Spirituality Itself or Consciousness Itself. Food-taking is simply a biological matter. Therefore, the effective taking of food has to do with matters of biology and the principles of the living system and its reactions.

The practice of right diet is a bodily discipline, not a Spiritual discipline. The practice of right diet originates (and, essentially, belongs) in the context of the first three stages of life—or the physical platform on which all of psycho-physically activated practice is done. The practice of right diet does not, itself, relate to the Transcendental Spiritual Process Itself. I Criticize all notions that have to do with physical (or psycho-physical, or conditional) seeking for some presumed-to-be-ultimate state—whether a Spiritual state or a state of extreme longevity or whatever.

Critical Address to Five Key Points

• Relative to any matter of discipline, Avatar Adi Da critically addresses five key points of egoic misunderstanding:

1. egoity

2. seeking

3. the "yes"/"no" extremes on either side of the basic requirements of intrinsically ego-transcending practice

4. stages-of-life prejudices (or any and all attachments to a particular developmental stage of life, and, also, to the characteristic illusions associated with that stage of life)

5. Great-Tradition* attachments (or even any and all uninspected presumptions, of any kind).

Each and all of My Instructions relative to the functional, practical, relational, and cultural disciplines of the only-by-Me Revealed and Given "Radical" Reality-Way of Adidam carry with Them a Critical Address to <u>five</u> key points: egoity, seeking, the "yes"/"no" extremes on either side of the basic requirements of intrinsically ego-transcending practice, stages-of-life prejudices (or any and all attachments to a particular developmental stage of life, and, also, to the characteristic illusions associated with that stage of life), and Great-Tradition attachments (or even any and all uninspected presumptions, of any kind). Each of those five key points is basic to My Instruction. Everyone has an orientation or a tendency, in some direction or other, that relates to these five key points. Therefore, My Address to right diet—and the address made to the dietary practice of My devotees by designated representatives of the cooperative cultural gathering

---

* The "Great Tradition" is Avatar Adi Da's term for the total "inheritance" of historical, "religious", and Spiritual paths and philosophies of humankind.

of My devotees—must speak not only to the "subject" of a particular functional, practical, relational, or cultural form of discipline, but must make reference to these five key points. Every form of My Instruction is an Argument That Addresses the egoic tendencies in people. This Address should Inspire people and Help them to correct themselves in their life-practice. And such understanding of My Instruction clearly identifies the Uniqueness of the Reality-Way of Adidam As My Divine Avataric Revelation. ■

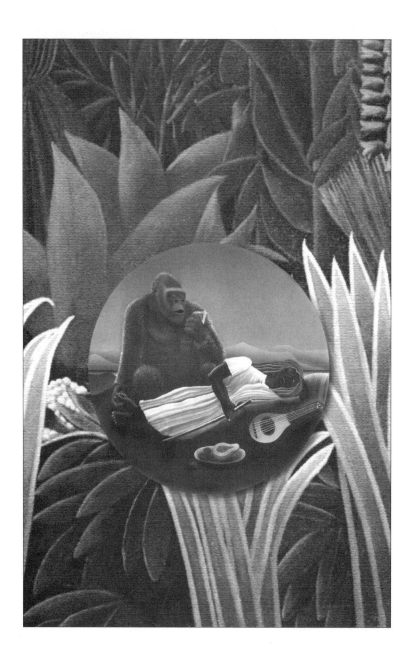

PART TWO

Discourses on
the Searchless Raw Diet

The Right-Life Discipline of Searchless Raw Diet and Fasting

1.

T he searchless raw diet is a basic right-life discipline in the Reality-Way of Adidam Ruchiradam. Therefore, that dietary discipline has a specific purpose, and a specific basis for determining the effectiveness of the discipline.

The dietary practice that I have Given My devotees is a raw-food diet. Apart from certain physical factors that may make a diet of exclusively raw food impractical in rare cases, the principle of the dietary discipline is that once the body is in a purified and balanced condition, then only food is taken that is necessary to sustain the body in its well-being and healthfulness. If you will observe that principle, then you will constantly be addressing all of the "self"-indulgent preferences of the body-mind-"self" that result in toxicity and imbalance, and you will practice a diet of raw food.

The common tendency relative to all aspects of ordinary life is not only to exercise egoic habits but to constantly reinforce in oneself and in others the principle of social "good feeling" as a solution to the stress of life. People are always encouraging one another, with their conventional social messages, to re-enter the play of social relations, because they feel it to be the right arrangement of life. Relative to diet, people commonly influence one another in all kinds of ways to embrace habits of taking things into the body. Thus, diet becomes a social practice to achieve social pleasure, ultimately to pleasurize the body for its own sake.

Someone who would practice the Reality-Way of Adidam might likewise achieve a mediocre resolution of diet in order to justify all kinds of habits of "self"-indulgence, with the justification that, as long as the diet is vegetarian and the person is not grossly overeating, he or she is practicing a version of the dietary discipline I have Given. That is simply not true. The glorification of the social ego to itself has nothing to do with the Reality-Way of Adidam. Nor is the practice of diet in the Reality-Way of Adidam merely idealistically vegetarian. All of that is simply a "lifestyle cop-out", a short-term diversion. The practice of diet I have Given is the intensive purifying and balancing of the body through maintaining a strict diet that supplies the body only the food that it requires for a continued pure and balanced state of physical well-being—meaning a body that has vitality and that has been made strong.

The principle of purifying and balancing the body, and keeping it in a purified and balanced state of well-being, is the basis for any nourishing of the body for the sake of its vitality. To abandon the pure and balanced bodily state and adhere to an idealized dietary practice is not to practice the dietary discipline that I have Given. You must first bring the body into a state of balance by correcting old habits and purifying the body of the results of old habits. Such purification includes fasting. When the body has achieved a purified and balanced state, then what is the dietary practice that sustains its vital well-being? That practice is a raw diet.

It is important for the body to be purified and balanced in order to effectively practice the dietary discipline as I have just described it. If, in the case of particular individuals, it is found (for right medical reasons) that the individual body cannot rightly be sustained by an exclusively raw diet, then the diet must, necessarily, be "maximally raw", and whatever food is added to the diet must not otherwise toxify and create imbalance in the body. My devotee practices the discipline of diet consistently and over time, and in that practice observes the signs that may be shown in the body. One does not simply practice the discipline of diet until an "ideal" diet (that is right under all circumstances) is achieved. There is no such unchanging "ideal" diet. The diet always requires some kind of adjustment in response to the body's signs.

The principle of right diet in the Reality-Way of Adidam is not that you must be inspired to be a consumer of a diet that is attractive and that sounds interesting. The dietary practice in the Reality-Way of Adidam is a right-life discipline that is embraced in obedience to Me in a life of devotional turning to Me. Therefore, it is about constantly doing what you must do, according to the Instructions that I have Given, to purify and balance the body and keep it that way.

In particular, the dietary practice involves your constant re-sensitization to the processes in the body. You must constantly measure the body's well-being and be aware, through disciplining the body, of the body's signs. You must bring the body into a state of purification and balance, and practice diet from day to day on that lawful basis. That pure and balanced condition is the lawfulness of the dietary practice. On that basis, and from day to day, you practice the diet that simply maintains the basic condition of purity and balance, taking into the body what is necessary from day to day for vital well-being, fundamental strength, and functionality of the body.

2.

People tend to think of fasting as a yearly (or regular, or periodic) purification. Actually, fasting is part of the dietary cycle. Fasting is purifying, yes, but it also rebalances the system. Fasting must be engaged intelligently, and there are many forms of fasting that are beneficial—taking one meal a day for several days, for example, or taking no food for twenty-four hours, or fasting with only liquids for a few or many days, and so on—using fasting in a rhythmic or responsibly random fashion. Really, fasting is a form of diet, and it should be regarded as part of the diet and not merely something you do instead of eating.

When the body shows particularly exaggerated signs of toxicity, then a long fast may be required. However, if you maintain the raw diet and take short fasts with some significant frequency, then an occasional extended fast of seven to ten days will perhaps be sufficient. You may even find that the body thrives on a liquid diet (fasting with juices). Few people, if anyone, can go without eating entirely, but frequent fasts may be beneficial, even for extended periods, as the body develops its fundamental balance and purified state.

Diet is a necessity. Fasting is more a natural condition. Whenever the body shows that diet is not necessary—for instance, if there is an aggravation in the body—then it is time to fast again. In some sense, truly, eating is an activity that you engage between fasts, rather than the other way around. Fasting is the natural condition of the body. Based on that understanding of the inherent wisdom of the body, eating is more the occasional necessity.

Recent investigations into longevity have identified three places in the world with the highest number of people per capita who live to be one hundred years old. The phenomenon is unique to these three places. The investigative studies conclude that two factors are unique to the centenarians in these places. One is that the levels of DHEA* in the centenarians in these regions have decreased more slowly than in the general population. The second factor is that the people in these three places have a tradition of systematically under-eating. They constantly—daily—introduce the principle

---

* Dehydroepiandrosterone (DHEA) is a natural steroid prohormone regarded as a precursor to sex steroids. Both regular exercise and caloric restriction have been shown to increase DHEA levels in the body, and some theorize that increased DHEA levels are at least partially responsible for the longer life-expectancy associated with caloric restriction.

of fasting by their particular practice of food-taking. The practice of systematic under-eating has long been identified as a healthful practice—whatever the form of one's diet might be, and before such elements as DHEA became known. Those who notice the principles that support longevity have long observed that under-eating is fundamental to health. It has long been recommended that one should eat less than you feel you want, without necessarily counting the calories or applying any other principles of diet.

Intelligence about fasting—in whatever form—is a physical understanding, and not a mental one. People who are bound by bodily dependencies that come from habit never realize this understanding. One must be willing to experiment with food-taking and fasting in order to determine how the body works.

The taking of food is a necessary burden on the body, so its effects must always be repaired by fasting. Fasting and taking food work together. When you are fasting and the body begins to show signs of depletion, it is time to be eating. Continue eating, then, until it is clear that you should be fasting again. As you apply the principles of the raw diet, you develop the sensitivity to the length of time and the rhythm of your fasting. You become sensitive to when you should fast and when you should eat again. Making use of this sensitivity allows optimum health for the body.

In fasting, there is a kind of natural freedom from much of the imposition of bodily existence. Much that people are suffering is rooted in how they treat the physical. The demands of the body for gross food, the burden of its diseases and mortality, and its cravings of all kinds can be brought into balance by the intelligent use of right diet and fasting.

The use of fasting is not a Spiritual matter. It is just another means for optimally disciplining the natural, or bodily, dimension, such that it is principled, rather than a phenomenon with which you must always struggle.

3.

The signs of a predisposition toward any kind of physical disorder in the body-mind-complex are observable in the body-mind-complex. When such signs are noticed, they should be taken seriously, before the aggravated and advanced symptoms appear. It tends to be the case, however, that people do not become serious about their health until they become ill.

Truly, the best way to deal with illness is to prevent illness, through the consistent practice of right life. The right-life practice in the Reality-Way of Adidam is effectively a preventative of all kinds of disorders that may (otherwise) develop over time. The discipline is not engaged for mere health reasons, but for the reason of right-life practice in the context of "radical" devotion to Me, which deals with the disposition and tendencies of an individual altogether.

Nevertheless, people tend to become serious about disciplining themselves only when they are at their worst, whereas they should be disciplining themselves at all times and under all conditions. People would be in a maximally healthful state, generally speaking, even all their lives, if they maintained the discipline of a raw diet—in other words, if they maintained a life-long discipline of diet instead of waiting until they feel unwell to become serious about diet and health and then, at that point, seeking to cure themselves.

The habits of life of people in their early years of adulthood show signs in the body like the rings in a tree. These life-habits generate effects in later life, in the years of middle to old age. Because of the variety of constitutions among people, the signs are different in everyone's case but nobody dies from nothing. Death comes from the burden that the body bears throughout a lifetime. In and of itself, longevity is not a virtue. The virtue is in the practice of right life, which in the later years of one's life is simply a continuation of one's practice of right-life discipline from an early age.

The right-life practice of health in the Reality-Way of Adidam positively optimizes the effects of habits of life, and it does so without any form of seeking-effort. Though countering the effects of unhealthful habits is not the purpose of the right-life discipline, nevertheless, such positive signs may be observed. People who maintain the practices of right life in the Reality-Way of Adidam are not attracted to the search for cure and the search for bodily well-being. They simply maintain the discipline of health without the exaggerations of seeking for it.

The dietary discipline in the Reality-Way of Adidam is not a cure. It is simply right life. Any approach that proposes a cure is the ego's search for consolation. The search for cure always comes about in response to the arising of a negative event in the bodily life. By contrast, My devotees are founded in the intelligent choice to practice right-life discipline because of their devotional response to Me. Secondarily, the practice of right life in the Reality-Way of Adidam is also preventive—and, therefore, curative in the sense that the practice of the right-life discipline of health is free from the egoic search.

I have, over all the years of My Work of Submission to Teach My devotees, proven the discipline of right life in My Own Body. Therefore, what is the right dietary practice? It is the consistent dietary practice of a raw diet.

Right life, maximum well-being, and the maintaining of a discipline throughout life that keeps the body consistently pure and balanced and vitalized and able to participate in the Way of Realization for which right life is the support—such is essential to right and true practice of the Reality-Way of Adidam Ruchiradam. ■

The Green Domain

1.

The raw diet that I recommend for My devotees is essentially a diet of fruits and greens. People try to compensate for the things that the raw diet does not include by taking, for example, large quantities of nuts and seeds, thereby creating an imbalanced diet that causes health problems. Because nuts and seeds are high in fat, which bothers the liver, they should be taken in moderation, if at all.

Finding a sustainable balance is the key to the practice of diet for My devotees. Nevertheless, fruits and greens are the fundamental constituents of the raw diet.

The so-called "green drinks" made of blended greens provide the balance of nutrition that an individual requires, and they do so efficiently—because to take as many greens as you need for a balanced raw diet you would have to spend all day eating salad.* The green drinks make the vegetables palatable as well, by the addition of a small amount of fruit, which adds a sweet flavor. Spirulina, chlorella, and wheatgrass may also be added.

The conventional meal generally emphasizes cuisine rather than principles. Therefore, anyone among My devotees who prepares raw food must become educated in the principles of the lawful use of raw food. The preparer of raw food should not try to emulate the conventional cook with the conventional cookbook in the conventional

---

* Please see section 5 in part three about "green drinks" (pp. 114–15). Avatar Adi Da also makes reference in this essay to research on greens presented in *Green for Life* and other publications listed in "For Further Study", pp. 130–34.

kitchen. Conventional methods of cookery are not appropriate to a raw diet. The raw diet is based on certain principles of health, on watching the body's signs and adjusting the diet accordingly.

In the Reality-Way of Adidam Ruchiradam, diet is medicine. Therefore, diet is to be practiced knowledgeably, in response to bodily signs and on the basis of the principles that I have Given. That which does the body good is a gift to the body that enables the body to cure itself and maintain its own balance and vitality. You would find the substances that do the body good if you were wandering in the wilderness. Because the wilderness is green, mainly your food would be green. Some things that plants bear are edible, such as the various kinds of seeds and even their flora, but most of any plant is green. If you were to maintain the diet based on the food you find while you are wandering through the woods, your diet would be mainly green.

The message to human beings from the natural world is this: Eat the green, and eat a little bit of the rest, and do not kill anybody in your effort to sustain yourself. Nuts, seeds, and fruits are part of the raw diet. Principally, however, there is the green. Blender drinks of many kinds of green (with a little bit of fruit to taste), some fruits, nuts and seeds, and sprouts (which are part of the green domain)—those are the essential elements of right diet in the Reality-Way of Adidam.

Some people presume raw diet to be an extreme kind of ascetical practice. However, the diet I recommend is just a practical discipline. Diet has nothing to do with Spiritual life as I describe it, except that the diet I recommend brings the body into conjunction with a right life practice that supports the, ultimately, Transcendental Spiritual process I Awaken in My devotees.

2.

Socrates is reported to have said, when he became an older man, that the worst of all the arts is cookery. Cooking uses the principle of fire to pander to "self"-indulgent and addictive tendencies. There is a fire in the yard or in the forest—the fire that Dylan Thomas called a "green fuse".* The life-process is also a fire. The human body surrounds a fire in the middle, a "pyre-amid", a fire in the midst, the fire of ingestion and health. The fire inside the body is the fire of the raw diet. It is the fire in the field, the life-fire. Take the food that the fire in the field produces, which is dominantly green, and ingest it directly. You need not make cuisine out of it. You simply must prepare it so that the body can relate to it directly and not spend vast amounts of time to take it in. Not fire and cookery, but blender technology is the best invention for diet.

The fruits or fruit juices that are added to make palatable the intense flavor of a green drink are part of the fruit dimension of the raw diet. The green dimension of the raw diet is the nourishing dimension. Some nourishment is gained from fruits, nuts, and seeds, but principally the diet is green. More than any other food, greens contain the fundamental requirements for health. No other food has the same level of sustaining chemistry that greens have. Greens contain the maximum necessary nourishment, more than any other form of food, including fruits and nuts and seeds. Therefore, greens are the principal diet for human beings.

* See Thomas's poem, "The Force that Through the Green Fuse Drives the Flower".

3.

In the world in general, there is not a great deal of understanding of the principles of such a diet. Over thirty years ago, I named My first book about diet *The Eating Gorilla Comes In Peace*. What do gorillas eat? What are the primates who are close to the human form doing? They are practicing a raw diet. They haven't a clue about how to build a fire and cook something. They move about, so that they are constantly foraging in different places and taking food from different sources. The gorilla's diet is dominantly greens. Secondarily, the diet of the gorilla makes use of various kinds of fruits and seeds.

Gorillas spend a tremendous amount of time every day in taking food. They do not have much to do otherwise, so they sit around and eat greens off the bushes. To chew and ingest such a diet takes time. Human beings, however, do not generally have the leisure to wander and forage. Most people would have to walk a long distance before they could find something green and edible that is growing in the wild. The activities of foraging and wandering and spending all day in eating are not practical for humankind.

The raw diet is something like an in-the-wild diet. However, in order to eliminate the amount of time you must spend at this diet, you must prepare the food in such a way that it is readily absorbed and that eating it does not require much time. Juices and blended preparations are a solution. These green drinks maintain the activity of eating that the body is built to do, which is to ingest greens in a daily cycle, not only to purify itself but to constantly rebuild, rebalance, and revitalize itself. The raw diet gives you the entire "pill"—purification and then rebalancing and then rebuilding and revitalizing.

If, like the gorilla, you take green leafy vegetables but in a concentrated form, the food is medicine, as the raw diet is meant to be, and you need not spend your life in eating. An added advantage is that the preparation of your food is not complicated—because the meal is not cuisine.

People who confess that they cannot fast readily or that they lose too much weight by fasting can practice this raw diet with green drinks every day and maintain their weight, even encourage the body to find its own weight. The raw diet with green drinks is not a weight-loss diet. It is not merely purifying. It is sustaining, and it provides what no other diet can provide, because all other forms of diet are several steps away from the nutritional sources that maximize the nutrition the body needs, causing the body to acquire toxins and to suffer imbalance and devitalization.

People who maintain the raw diet in the form I recommend have less need for extended fasting, because the diet is naturally purifying, like a fast. Fasting is useful for other reasons, primarily to give the body a "vacation" from ingestion. Periodic fasting likewise serves the emotions and the mind.

There is really only one approach to right diet, and that is a diet of raw and (fundamentally) green food. The principal dietary practice in the Reality-Way of Adidam is a diet of raw greens in liquid form, taken three or more times per day, with other raw foods eaten in more or less whole form. A mis-application of the principles of raw diet emphasizes the purification phase of the body's process of taking food. People become weakened by a diet that mis-applies the principles of taking raw food. Then they try to compensate for the weakness by taking large quantities of seeds and nuts and the like, for starch and protein. That approach is the reason that people feel the raw diet does not work for them.

The right food for humankind is not anything that arrived on Earth after the plant domain established its universality in the Earth-world. The raw diet of green plants is right and lawful. Therefore, I call those who practice the Reality-Way of Adidam to maintain that fundamental dietary practice—and I also recommend that dietary practice to all of humankind.

Some people who are seriously ill may require remedial help because they might not be strong enough even to endure the process of the initial purification associated with sustaining the body with leafy greens and fruit. Exceptions can be made for people with such unique medical requirements. However, all My devotees who can responsibly maintain their lives and their diet choose the approach of an exclusively raw diet.

The raw diet is not overly sweet, and it is not merely purifying. It is a means for nourishing and constantly rebuilding and revitalizing the body—the body is constantly balanced. If you provide the body with the necessary food, the body balances itself. Nothing outside the body keeps the body in balance. The body systematically balances itself, when its cooperation with the natural domain is supported.

However, through all kinds of aberrated notions, the human mind tends to control the substances that the body is given to eat. The ego-mind not only destroys the body, but it destroys the world eventually, as is being demonstrated in this generation now. In this "dark" time, human beings are destroying the Earth-world itself, after centuries of the destruction of their own bodies.

Human beings are addicts—ego-bound, and seeking to "feel good". They must unlearn—and they must be willing to unlearn—their addictions, and they must be governed rightly through right education and accountability. The propagandizing of activities that do harm to humankind must be undermined, whereas such activities now cover the Earth.

4.

It is known that in the "green world", the birds and insects that distribute the seeds constantly move about and create a vast variety of green life. It is also known that every green form contains a minute amount of some form of alkaloid, which is a poison. Every growing green thing contains alkaloid in minute amounts and of a particular kind. Every growing green thing contains its own kind of alkaloid to make the non-humans who feed on it sick such that they will move on to some other form of green. By these means the process of reproduction continues in a world of vast variety.

Therefore, new genetic influences are constantly appearing. The various creatures that carry the seeds ingest the green thing and then eliminate it somewhere else. Such is the strategy of survival in the natural world. All natural forms are involved in that very pursuit of complexity for the sake of their survival.

If you take just one kind of green long enough, eventually you will no longer want to have it. You will have accumulated too much of the particular poison in that green, and you will feel unwell. However, do not then stop taking greens. Instead, take another kind of green. You must constantly vary the greens that you take. A principal leaf form could be taken for a while, and then you must change to another leaf form so as not to accumulate too much of the homeopathic dose of toxin that is in the particular green you are having at the moment.

The fact that the green contains an alkaloid toxin is not negative. It is simply something to understand in order to maintain variety while still taking an all-green preparation. Look out the door. Look at all the variety. The green world is not all one thing, not just a single green blade sticking up in the air. A myriad of green leaves exists. That world of variety exists because of the method of distribution that underlies the natural domain.

The inventiveness of human commerce allows human beings access to all kinds of sources, such that people today are not merely taking food that is raised in the local area. Today there is dietary variety through commerce that provides sources of food from places at a distance.

The green world was the first to "colonize" the Earth, and everything else came afterward. All other life-forms are derived from the green world and are dependent on it. A dimension of the problem in the world today is the destruction of the green domain. Human beings have interfered with cosmic Nature and are paying the price—are about to pay a terrible price if they do not reverse this trend, if they do not understand the lesson, restore the green domain, and live on the gift of the green domain instead of destroying it and the animals that participate in its method of distribution.

5.

In ancient times, people sacrificed animals to a sacred domain that they presumed surrounded or was otherwise inaccessible to the human world. The sacrifice of animals to make a connection from humans to the energy-world, or the spirit-world, became a widespread practice in the ancient religions.

Even vegetarianism in the ancient world was, in part, a revolt against the sacrifice of animals and against the temple practices that were otherwise current in the society. By practicing vegetarianism, someone could demonstrate disagreement with the religious practices of the society at large at the time. Thus, vegetarianism was a kind of underground practice. It was unorthodox. Someone who practiced vegetarianism was not just frowned upon but could even be punished for it.

People sacrifice animals in their own guts now on a constant basis. Vast industries for the slaughter of animals exist all over the world. The industry for processing animal products for sacrifice in the temple of the human body is one of the major forms, if not the principal form, of aggravation of the natural world that is producing global warming. The murder of animals for this purpose is a practice against which human beings should revolt. However, it is being held in place by the industries of advertising and junk foods. People are being duped by these industries into maintaining the practice of taking killed food—and people are ill.

The temple practices of the ancient world have been universalized to the extent that people all over the earth are maintaining themselves for the most part on animal slaughter, blood-letting for the satisfying of human addiction. The temple of today's world is a different kind of temple—it is the temple of the ego, the temple of the stomach. Animals are raised under industrial circumstances of terrible suffering, and they are murdered, sacrificed, and thrown into the guts of human beings, who are creating problems in the balance of the Earth now with this practice and with various other addictive practices in which they indulge—and these same human beings are constantly unwell.

Effectively a revolution is required in the human world to prevent human beings from destroying the human race and the Earth itself. Humankind must be restored to Truth, to right understanding, and to right practice of life. Therefore, not only restoration of the planet but right dietary practice must be advocated. The restoration of the planet's balance is absolutely appropriate advocacy and a necessary change. Nevertheless, there must also be a change in human practice relative to the matters of human health.

Diet is a principal form of the human connection to the larger world, and it is simply true that the "green domain" of plants is the natural source of food for human beings. The social and political concern about global warming and climate change is connected to matters of diet. The industrialization of the raising of animals in order to kill them for food is a gross violation of the natural laws of responsibility that are incumbent upon human beings. Not only is the animal industry a dreadful abuse of non-humans, but it is also contaminating the atmosphere on the same scale as emissions from the burning of fossil fuels.

Right practice of health is essentially a matter of giving up one's addictions, which are always ego-based, and adhering to a right diet, which is a green diet. Re-green the Earth, but eat green too. Do not kill animals anymore. Abandon the murderous disposition toward the living world of self-conscious beings. Do not indulge in dietary addictions. Restore a source of pure food by restoring the pure, green world.

6.

A raw, dominantly green diet is not simply good for your health. That raw, green diet is lawful. To adhere to the raw, dominantly green diet is right life in the greatest sense of lawful participation in the Earth-world and the universe.

People tend not to know what is lawful. They do not know the principles of living in this dimension of appearances. This Earth-world is not utopia by any means, and cannot be. Nevertheless, there is a lawful way to live here and participate in the Divine Reality. There is a lawful way to serve the situation of humankind through the practice of transcending egoity, transcending bondage to this or any form of appearances. There is a lawfulness of life—and I am Communicating it here.

The traditional messages point to it, but those communications also have their limitations. My Reality-Teaching is the Truth of Reality Itself, Which Is Divine. It is simply, straightforwardly, Purely Given. It has been brought to humankind at Great Cost. A Great Submission was required of Me, even to be able to bring the Communication of Truth through this Body. My Life Time has been a Great Submission to human beings in order to test the Truth in the context of human life.

All that has had to be done by Me, and My Reality-Teaching is complete, Addressing all issues in a complete and summary fashion. Matters of diet, including health, simply have to do with the process of living in the apparently material, conditional universe, and in the Earth-world as it appears in human experience. For many years, My devotees have had My Instruction about raw diet, fully Given by Me as their obligation. Even from the earliest days of My Teaching-Work, I constantly advocated dietary practice in dialogue with My devotees, and I Called them to experiment with many dietary approaches. I did not invent the raw diet, but I am advocating it. Yet the greater purpose of My Divine Avataric Appearance here is not to tell people about raw diet. Right practice of diet is an entirely ordinary matter, a form of discipline to be established in the foundation stages of the Reality-Way of Adidam Ruchiradam. ■

Searchless, Lawful Management
of the Body

1.

Someone who rightly practices diet and fasting in the manner I recommend naturally enjoys physical well-being. Someone who exploits diet for pleasure has fun and then suffers. You may choose one or the other approach to life. You can have fun and suffer, or you can enjoy a continuous sense of well-being and enjoy freedom from the negative exaggerations of physical existence.

Fun and suffering are two sides of a self-replicating cycle. People who embrace the conventions of the social world in order to maximize fun and pleasure inevitably must struggle with mortality, disease, and bodily stresses. Most such people cannot even imagine living a principled physical existence in which they are naturally free of the cycle of pleasure, disease, and suffering. Ultimate Freedom, Transcendental Spiritual Freedom, is something else again, a Spiritual matter. Yet the natural bodily freedom of which I speak may be enjoyed by anyone. The usual person does not, in general, embrace the disciplining that bodily well-being requires unless he or she has no choice, having become so physically degraded as to be forced to change his or her habit of life. Only then does such a person choose to live—at least to a degree—in such a manner as to become healthy.

It is possible, however, to choose the lawful physical practice all your life. By tendency, people break out of such a practice into the fun-and-suffering worldliness that is everywhere propagandized in their society. Yet within a culture of practice of right life and physical well-being, every person is an example and an encouragement for every other person, an inspiration to lawful practices of all kinds, the practice of right life (including diet and health) as well as Spiritual life. Well-being should be the sign in such a culture of inspiration and expectation, a culture that transcends the dramatizing of reluctance to discipline the body-mind-"self" and the constant fascination with the results of an unprincipled life. In the culture of the "Radical" Reality-Way of Adidam (or Adidam Ruchiradam), right life is practiced, and the signs are shown in every person, for all to observe.

In a merely social gathering, people seek to preserve egoity and the habits of suffering. Listen to what people say. What do they constantly inspire in one another? The exploitation of egoity and the life of bondage to the body and the "world". The speech of every person in conventional society is propaganda. Good company, or the company of those who inspire and expect the practice of right life in one another, is fundamental to the practice of the Reality-Way of Adidam. Bad company does not so inspire. Generally speaking, people who are governed by the ego are bad company. Such people encourage one another toward a life that may seem attractive, but its attractiveness is only temporary and soon disappears.

Traditionally, it is said that the best thing that one can do is to spend time in the Company of the Realizer, the Master, and to live within the Master's Sphere—in other words, to live in the good company of those who practice devotion, right life, and Spiritual practice in the Company of the Master. Not only is the Master's Company the place of Spiritual Transmission, of Which the Master is the Source, but also in the Master's Sphere everyone exemplifies the Way of right life and encourages one another in the Way of right life and responds to one another's signs, thereby keeping one another accountable for the Way of right life that is Given by the Master. In the "worldly" circumstance, on the other hand, no such process of good company exists, even though the notion of the "good life" may be proposed and offered with smiles.

2.

If the body (in combination with the natural bodily energy) is established in a lawful position through diet, the body will (generally speaking) heal itself. Some assistance may be necessary to apply, over time, to bodily conditions that are resistive to self-healing. In such cases, essentially natural—and, basically, dietary means—may be applied. However, when one presumes that the body is a "problem" to be "solved", rather than a system to be lawfully managed, then exaggerated and systematic efforts to "cure" the body only interfere with the body's self-healing ability.

Therefore, not only is there a right diet in the Reality-Way of Adidam, but also there is a right Teaching to be understood about the practice of health. That right Teaching is the <u>searchless</u> application of diet.

This present book is, therefore, quite thin—because it does not describe a cuisine, nor explain dietary principles in scientific language, nor offer dietary "cures" that propose to heal the body from without, rather than simply supporting the lawful management of the body.

Managing the body lawfully is not—and should not be— a search. Managing the body lawfully is simply a principle of right life. Trying to "cure" the body by adding certain foods or supplements to the diet in the attempt to make the body well is seeking, and not the principle of right diet that I recommend.

For instance, if anyone has signs of disease, those signs should obviously be monitored and the changes in the body observed. Yet what is there to do otherwise? Maintain a lawful bodily state. And what is that lawful condition? Through the practice of right-life obedience to Me, in a life of devotional and moment to moment turning to Me, the lawful condition of the body-mind-complex is to be discovered and its principles understood.

The lawful bodily state is established and maintained through the application of a diet of raw food, the practice of which is founded in the principle of no-seeking. As a general rule, if the body is established in a lawful position, the body (in conjunction with its natural energies) will righten itself. Therefore, in the Reality-Way of Adidam, the discipline of diet establishes the "position" of well-being of the body, and the practice of diet is not an exaggerated address to, or manipulation of, the body.

The healing arts of both naturopathy and allopathy have a role to play when conditions in the body are resistive to that kind of self-healing. It must be understood, however, that the conventional ego-based and search-bound approach to healing assumes that people are patients to whom all manner of "cure" must be applied. That approach is a conventional approach that is both ego-bound and bound by the search. By contrast, the right practice of well-being is based on a Transcendental Spiritual understanding. This is My Communication. Even when people otherwise recommend natural diet, they are not necessarily approaching diet with a true Transcendental Spiritual understanding (even if they think they are doing so). In general, even otherwise healthful dietary recommendations are dictated by the conventional, search-bound orientation and state of those who recommend them.

Gross and ego-bound views manifest in all kinds of ways, organizing themselves through notions of "problem" and "search". Right diet in the Reality-Way of Adidam is not based in "problem" and "search". Right diet in the Reality-Way of Adidam is based in lawfulness. Fundamentally, it is the practice of assuming that you do not have a problem of health. Rather, you have an obligation for health, and not a problem to be corrected. When the body's functioning is limited in any way, yield the body to the lawful situation in which the condition may be set right, rather than presuming a problem and seeking a solution.

The practice of right diet in the Reality-Way of Adidam is a searchless practice—not a search for cure. The search for cure through diet—whether a raw diet or any other systematic approach to diet—is a fascinated preoccupation of many people in the present day. In the Reality-Way of Adidam, however, diet is simply an ordinary practice and an aspect of the larger practice of right-life discipline.

The first approach to all health issues is always to self-responsibly correct the body and apply lawful right discipline to it. Part of the process of the practice of right life in the Reality-Way of Adidam is time—one establishes the lawful practice and then allows the body time to show its signs. The process of right life is allowed to unfold, because through right discipline the body's energies have been set free to show their lawful signs. However, the lawful practice of diet, and of health altogether, is a process of observation and examination, and is not necessarily spontaneously corrective of all health issues. The healing arts are an important aid to the body if resistive conditions are still observed in the body over time.

The obsessive and fanatical seeking-approach that looks for magic cures is not the approach I give to My devotees in the Reality-Way of Adidam. If there is to be well-being, the body must be yielded to its unified circumstance in the unity of its natural domain. How is that yielding accomplished? Simply by establishing the lawfulness of bodily discipline. The body is a food-process. In the traditions of India, the body is called the "food body". Fundamentally, it does not need to be cured. One needs simply to stop bothering the body with "self"-indulgent habits of life, stop throwing it out of balance, stop maintaining it unlawfully.

The principle of "searchlessness" relative to diet and well-being is unique to My Instruction to My devotees. I have Criticized seeking in all its forms since the first day of My formal Work of Teaching. Therefore, My Criticism of seeking applies to all the searches for cure, and all the fanaticism relative to diet that may be found in today's marketplace.

People are always ready to work on their "problem", whatever it might be. In reality, you are your own "problem", and that is why you are always functioning as if you have one. The problem-free—or searchless—approach to discipline, rather than the search for a solution to a problem, is the principle of right-life practice in the Reality-Way of Adidam. This is not to imply that healing effects do not appear in the body when the principles of right diet are applied. Yes, healing may occur, but not because you have found the magic substance, the secret ingredient, for which you are always seeking. When you accept the discipline of lawfulness that I describe, healing is a spontaneous manifestation of the bodily life. Fundamentally, you leave the body alone. You observe its signs, rather than trying to manipulate it into well-being.

3.

The only-by-Me Revealed and Given Reality-Way of Adidam Ruchiradam is the Way of living differently. The Reality-Way of Adidam is the practice and the realization of principled well-being and freedom from ego-bondage. The disciplines of right life that are Given by Me in the Reality-Way of Adidam are embraced by My devotee in devotional recognition of Me and responsive devotional turning to Me. The practice of the Reality-Way of Adidam is right-life obedience to Me, and not merely a program for changes in one's lifestyle. The life-disciplines that I have Given are modes of a life that is lived on the foundation of principles that counter the ego-bondage of the ordinary "world".

The principles of right life in the Reality-Way of Adidam are not merely moral principles, although they certainly have moral force. The principles of right life in the Reality-Way of Adidam govern the domain of "money, food, and sex" and social egoity, such that the life of seeking to have fun and then suffering afterward—and cumulatively and more and more, and becoming more and more physically, emotionally, and mentally out of balance—is countered by maintaining principles of right life. The Reality-Way of Adidam is associated with principled right living, principled well-being, living by principles that demonstrate well-being, and living free—free of bondage to the cycle of fun and suffering, the search to be pleasurized and to avoid pain, the search for pleasure and the inevitable resultant suffering of pain. Therefore, the Reality-Way of Adidam is the abandoning of the egoic "method" of the "worldly" life. The cues one receives constantly from the "world" propagandize everyone into the life of pleasure and pain, fun and suffering. Everybody everywhere in the "world" is barraged with this propaganda by the hucksters of ordinary life everywhere—of which everybody is also one, essentially, to every "other". Every ego is a huckster, encouraging every other ego to join the ego-"world" and have some fun.

The Reality-Way of Adidam is a counter to the propaganda of the ego's "world". Right life is a life founded in the principles for living that manifest well-being. If you are to enjoy such well-being, you must maintain "self"-discipline. The practice of "self"-discipline is difficult for one who is already "self"-indulgent. The more "self"-indulgent you are, and the less principled, the more difficult it is to bring the body-mind to a disciplined condition. Once you have accomplished well-being, however, then the life based on the principles of "self"-discipline is relatively easy, certainly straightforward to maintain.

In the Reality-Way of Adidam My devotee embraces principles of right-life management, in devotional obedience to Me. My devotee proves his or her practice of right life by demonstrating well-being. If well-being is not manifested to the maximum through one's principled practice of right-life obedience to Me, then the person is not practicing rightly.

Simultaneous with the rightly managed life, with right-life practice, with principled right living, there is, intrinsically, freedom in the domain of the body-mind-"self". The practice relinquishes ego-bondage and the indulgence of life as an ego, or indulgence in the exploitation of "money, food, and sex" and social egoity. All these dimensions of ordinary life are subject to disciplines through right-life obedience to Me, until well-being is demonstrated and, coincident with that well-being, there is intrinsic human freedom.

To live a life in accordance with the principles of right-life discipline is itself a kind of freedom. Such a life is priorly free of the identification with bondage and with the "world"-mummery of the propaganda of fun and suffering, pleasure and pain. The devotional practice of the Reality-Way of Adidam is intrinsically ego-transcending. The right-life practice of obedience to Me is intrinsically a demonstration of well-being and freedom in the domain of the body-mind-"self".

Perfect Freedom is a matter of Transcendental Spiritual and Divine Self-Realization. Yet at the foundation of Divine Self-Realization is whole-bodily devotional turning to Me and right-life obedience to Me that demonstrates well-being. My devotee turns to Me—with whole bodily devotion and moment to moment—thereby demonstrating constant searchless Beholding of Me, and, on that basis, Transcendental Spiritual Communion with Me.

Such is the process of the Reality-Way of Adidam as a whole. At the foundation of the Reality-Way of Adidam is the establishment of whole bodily devotional turning to Me and right-life obedience to Me—meaning the application of principles of right life that demonstrate psycho-physical well-being and freedom from ego-bondage through intrinsically ego-transcending and devotional whole-bodily turning to Me. ■

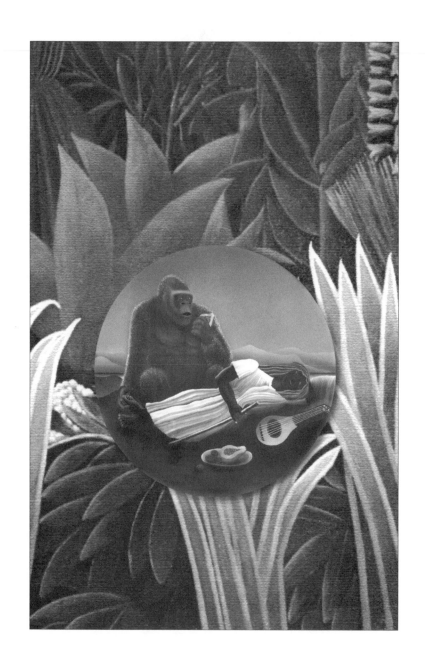

PART THREE

Living the Searchless
Raw Diet

Compiled by Members of the Radiant Life Clinic

1.

The Three Phases of the Health Process—
Purification, Rebalancing, and Rejuvenation

In the following excerpt from *The Dawn Horse Testament*, His Divine Presence Ruchira Avatar Adi Da Samraj provides a summary overview of the three phases of searchless (or "radical") health and healing: (1) purification, (2) rebalancing, and (3) rejuvenation. These phases are naturally supported by the lawful practice of right diet. Note that the many other practices of the Reality-Way of Adidam Ruchiradam that are mentioned in the following excerpt are defined briefly in the glossary and discussed at length in *The Dawn Horse Testament* as well as in *The Eating Gorilla Comes In Peace* and *Conscious Exercise and The Transcendental Sun.**

About the Radiant Life Clinic

The Radiant Life Cultural and Health Services (also known, more simply, as "The Radiant Life Clinic") was called into being by Ruchira Avatar Adi Da Samraj in 1979. Its principal responsibilities to Avatar Adi Da, His gathering of devotees, and the general public are to provide education, publications, and research. Health practitioners who are members of the Radiant Life Clinic also provide clinical and healing services. Individuals provide these services as Avatar Adi Da's devotees, in conformity with His Instructions relative to the "right life" principles Given by Avatar Adi Da Samraj. ∎

---

* New editions forthcoming from the Dawn Horse Press.

Phase of Health Process	Functional System of Body
Purification	Circulatory system
Rebalancing	Nervous system
Rejuvenation	Endocrine system

I n The Process Of "Radical" (or Fundamental and "At-The-Root") Healing, the Total bodily human being Is Addressed In Each Of The Three Phases. In Addition, Each Phase Also Particularly Addresses a specific functional system of the body. The First (or Purification) Phase Of The Process Of "Radical" Healing Purifies the circulatory system of the blood. The Second (or Rebalancing) Phase Balances The Two Halves Of the nervous system. And The Third (or Rejuvenation) Phase Regenerates the endocrine (or hormonal) system.

In Traditional Systems Of Health Practice, the blood Is Regarded As Corresponding To (or Representing) the etheric body—or The etheric Dimension Of the Total body-mind-complex. The emotional condition of the body-mind-complex Directly Affects the energy of the etheric body, Including the energy of the bodily-based being In General—and the blood Is The Basic Manifestation Of The Faculty Of emotion (or feeling). In its usual condition, the body-mind-complex Contracts emotionally—and The Resulting emotional Obstructions Have Their physical Counterparts In the organs of the body. The Processes Of Assimilation and Elimination Are Interrupted—and, Instead Of Simply Being Nourished Through The Process Of breathing and eating, the body Is Made toxic (Primarily, By the Obstructed emotional condition of the body-mind-complex).

First Phase of Healing = Purification

Participate in this phase via:

- Devotional Communion with Avatar Adi Da

- Abandoning contracted or reactive emotion, engaging free feeling-attention

- Engaging a purifying raw fructo-vegetarian diet

- Fasting

- Adequate rest

- Avoiding aggressive, motivated, and reactive behavior

- Right physical exercise

Therefore, The First Phase Of Healing, and The First Phase Of Maintaining General Health and Well-being, Is Purification—A Process That Includes Abandoning The Contracted Disposition Of emotion, Ceasing To Focus attention On emotional disturbances (and, Instead, Engaging The Fundamental Practice Of Intrinsically ego-Surrendering, ego-Transcending, and ego-Forgetting Devotional Communion With Me), Engaging A Purifying (and, Thus, raw fructovegetarian) Diet, Engaging Periodic (or, Otherwise, Therapeutic) Fasting, and Taking Adequate Rest. Instead Of Indulging In Aggressive, Motivated, and Reactive Behavior, Be Free Of emotional disturbances. Engage the body, In A Relaxed Disposition, Through Specific (Non-Strenuous) physical Exercises That Allow The Process Of Purification To Take Place In A Natural, Easeful Manner. This Is The First Phase Of Healing and The First Dimension Of The ordinary Maintaining Of General Health and Well-being.

Second Phase of Healing = Rebalancing

Participate in this phase via:

• Meditation

• Sacred activity

• "Conscious exercise"

• Pranayama

• "General conductivity" practice

• Yogic "conductivity" massage

• Use of hamsadanda and/or polarity screens, as well as other therapeutic modalities and/or devices that have a rebalancing effect on the body

• All forms of functional, practical, and relational "self"-discipline

The "two halves of the nervous system" that must be balanced are the sympathetic and the parasympathetic, which are both part of the autonomic nervous system. The autonomic nervous system is the part of the nervous system that is generally understood not to be typically controlled by conscious thought or intention.

The sympathetic nervous system, which is sometimes referred to as the "fight or flight" mechanism, is responsible for priming the body for action. The parasympathetic nervous system, which is sometimes referred to as the "rest and digest" mechanism, conserves energy as it slows the heart rate, increases intestinal and gland activity, and relaxes muscles in the gastrointestinal tract. The synergistic function of these two halves of the nervous system is crucial to maintaining dynamic equilibrium in the body—which is part of what Avatar Adi Da means relative to the "balancing" of the nervous system.

(continued in box on next page)

Sympathetic Nervous System System	Parasympathetic Nervous Nervous SystemSystem
"fight or flight"	"rest and digest"
bodily action	digestion and elimination
energy expenditure	energy conservation

The disciplines that Avatar Adi Da has given to balance the two halves of the autonomic nervous system directly affect the so-called non-volitional aspects of the being. The ability to affect the equilibrium of the body in this way has been known since ancient times in traditional cultures, but Western science is only beginning to acknowledge this through experiments measuring the impact of such practices as meditation, bio-feedback, and so on. ■

The Second Phase Of Healing, and The Second Phase Of Maintaining General Health and Well-being, Is The Process Of Balancing The Two Halves Of the nervous system. The Regime That Serves This Process Of Rebalancing Includes Meditation . . . , The Various By-Me-Given Forms Of Sacred Activity, "Conscious Exercise", Pranayama, "General Conductivity" Practice, Yogic "Conductivity" Massage, and (Altogether) All The Forms Of functional, practical, and relational "self"-Discipline I Describe. . . . These By-Me-Given Practices May Also (As Appropriate and Necessary) Be Supported By The Use Of The Hamsadanda and/or Polarity Screens, As Well As Other Therapeutic Modalities and/or Devices That Have A Rebalancing Effect On the body.

Third Phase of Healing = Rejuvenation

• Regenerated endocrine chemistry should be naturally produced by the body itself once purification and re-balancing are established.

• Conservation and re-circulation of sexual energy supports this energizing chemistry.

The Third Phase Of Healing, and The Third Phase Of Maintaining General Health and Well-being, Is The Intensification Of Available bio-physical energy (or Natural life-energy, or nerve-force) In the body-mind-complex, which Has Now Been Prepared To Receive (and Make Use Of) Such energy By Virtue Of The Purification and Rebalancing Phases Of The Process Of Healing. The Regenerated endocrine chemistry Should Be Naturally Produced By the body (itself). Therefore, Optimally, Such chemistry Is Not Introduced From Without. As A Matter Of The daily Maintenance Of Good Health and Well-being, The Processes Of Purification and Rebalancing Are (In and Of Themselves) Generally Sufficient To Prepare the body To Produce A More Benign Level Of chemistry (Of The Non-Stress Variety). Also, Among The Specific Practices That Contribute To The Introduction Of this Energizing chemistry and nerve-force In the body-mind-complex Is The Conservation and Re-Circulation Of sexual energy and its chemistry, In "Emotional-Sexual Devotional Communion" (or, Otherwise, "Emotional-Sexual Conscious Exercise") and, Also, In The "Own-Body Yogic Sexual Practice".

All Healing, and The Maintaining Of Optimum General Health and Well-being, Depends Upon This Three-Part Cycle (Of Purification, Rebalancing, and Rejuvenation). Therefore, Maintain Your Practice For The General Health Of the body-mind-complex In A Manner That Adheres To These Laws Of bodily Existence. Maintaining A Purifying (raw fructo-vegetarian) Diet, A Right (Non-toxifying) emotional Disposition, and A General psycho-physical Regime That Balances the body-mind-complex Will (In The General Case) Be Sufficient To Stimulate the endocrine system To Constantly Regenerate Natural life-energy and Maintain Optimum General Health and Well-being.

The Logic Of The Three-Part Cycle (Of Purification, Rebalancing, and Rejuvenation) Is Significant Not Only For The Process Of Healing but Also For The Process Whereby Optimum General Health Is Maintained (Once It Has Been Achieved).

While the optimal raw dietary practice supports all three phases of the health process, conscious food-taking is most fundamentally related to the first, or purification, phase of health and well-being. Therefore, one of the primary purposes of right diet is to purify the body, by eliminating any toxic build-up that would prevent a balanced and regenerated physical state.

2.
Intelligent Dietary Transitions

Bringing intelligence to any dietary change is crucial, and the transition to the searchless raw diet especially requires an approach that manages the necessary purification of accumulated toxins in the body and is established on the basis of an ongoing understanding of your own body's needs on the raw diet. Such transition should also be engaged in the problem-free disposition of Communion with the Living Reality, so that it does not become a goal-oriented or obsessive aspect of life. Avatar Adi Da summarizes His Instruction about dietary adaptation and transition:

> *In making an intelligent approach to dietary practice, it is critically important that you rightly manage the transition from a conventional (or "worldly") diet to the raw fructo-vegetarian diet—otherwise, your unpreparedness will likely lead you to feel that the by-Me-Given dietary principles do not work in your case. . . .*
>
> *Refine (or simplify) your diet progressively, and, thus (but as directly and quickly as possible), pass through the necessary cycles of purification, rebalancing, and rejuvenation— until, in the course of Second Congregation practice of the Reality-Way of Adidam (or, otherwise, in the course of dietary adaptation engaged by any individual), the discipline of "minimum optimum" (and, as a general rule, <u>totally</u> raw) diet (in the manner that has been demonstrated to be right and appropriate in your particular case, including the appropriately alternated cycles of purification, rebalancing, and rejuvenation, and with food taken always in minimum, but adequate, quantities) is <u>stably</u> achieved. . . .*
>
> *The total transition from conventional (or "worldly") dietary practice to practice of right "minimum optimum" (and, as a general rule, <u>totally</u> raw) diet is a matter of a*

properly planned (and, as necessary, even medically supervised) transitional process of functional (and even mental and emotional) adaptation. As a general rule, the course of dietary adaptation should readily and quickly proceed from basic fructo-vegetarian dietary practice to a totally raw fructo-vegetarian dietary practice (consisting principally of greens and fruits—with intensive daily use of "green drinks").

As a general rule, the process of adaptation to a fructo-vegetarian (fruit-and-vegetable) dietary practice that is consistently totally raw may rightly take from several weeks to between one and two months (or, in rare cases, even longer), with the actual transition-time determined by the previous habits, the strength of intention, and the general state of health of the individual. And, in <u>every</u> case, that practice-demonstration (or, otherwise, the right practice-demonstration of any medically necessary variation on the "minimum optimum" diet), when it is right and real and true, is always (and necessarily) associated with profound and life-practice-converting discoveries about the body-mind-"self"—such that further practice-demonstration in the Reality-Way of Adidam is (thereby) given an extraordinarily positively transformed psycho-physical basis.

—His Divine Presence
Ruchira Avatar Adi Da Samraj
(pp. 48, 37, 42–43)

Dietary Transition Via Fasting

Avatar Adi Da's principal recommendation relative to transition to the searchless raw diet is to prepare for and engage an extended fast, including at least some period of lemon-water fast. Such an extended fast not only purifies the body of accumulated toxins and re-balances the body, but also interferes with the repetitive habit-cycles of addictive tendencies relative to eating. In the wake of such a fast, the transition to raw diet is less of a struggle and becomes, instead, a response to discovering what is more natural, or native, to the body.

To make use of the fasting transition to the raw diet, you must first engage preparation for the fasting phase:

1. Remove the Most Toxic Elements of the Diet

• First relinquish use of stimulating foods and accessories to the diet—including alcohol and other addictive drugs (street or prescription), cigarettes, caffeinated drinks (coffee, black tea, sodas, "energy" drinks, etc.), white sugar and other sugar products, and excessive use of salt. Some may find relinquishing these foods and accessories straightforward, adapting over a period of a few days or weeks. Others may take longer for various reasons.

• Blended green drinks (see pp. 114–15) will assist the body in this and all phases of dietary transition. Start with 10–16 oz. (300–475 ml) of green drink once a day and move to 32–64 oz. (1–2 quarts/1–2 liters) divided over two to three drinks a day (or possibly in one period, as you are moved).

• We advise those on medications to consult with their doctor(s) before they begin the transition phase to the raw diet—and also while living the raw diet—as to whether they still need some or all of their medications, or less of them. Over time most (or, in some cases, potentially all) medications may cease to be necessary as the conditions that they are prescribed for are relieved or corrected by the raw diet. However, this is not necessarily so and therefore should be determined in consultation with the appropriate doctor(s). It is also very important not to stop certain medications suddenly, as suddenly stopping some medications can cause severe problems. It is strongly advised that those on medication be in close touch with their doctor(s) relative to adjusting or ceasing their medications and not arbitrarily or independently stop (whether suddenly or slowly) some or all medications.

• The elimination of toxins will generally initiate a cycle of bodily purification. (See the section "Managing Symptoms of Purification", pp. 101–103.) Symptoms of purification generally can pass without a lot of concern or attention. If any symptoms persist or are of concern, consult with a qualified doctor or therapist.

• Assist the process of purification and adaptation with appropriate amounts of pure water (generally take up to 8 oz. [240 ml] of water eight times per day), good bowel habits (including the possible use of fiber such as psyllium husks, ground flaxseed, etc.), and exercises that emphasize stretching, whole-bodily feeling, and full breath.

2. Eliminate Animal Products

• Once the initial purification has passed from removing the most toxic and/or addictive substances from one's diet, begin to eat a principally plant-based diet, decreasing cooked food, and eliminating all animal protein, meats, fowl, fish, eggs, and dairy. Continue the green drinks and increase raw foods. This phase of transition may take only a few days or may take longer.

3. Eliminate Grains and Concentrated Fats

• Now eliminate cooked grains and concentrated fats (such as oils, nuts and nut butters, avocados, etc.) while continuing the green drinks. This transition should only take a few days.

4. Final Preparation for Fast: Fully Raw

• Spend one to three days before your fast eating the fully raw fructo-vegetarian diet, consisting primarily of greens (including 1–2 quarts [1–2 liters] of blended green drink per day) and fruits, with some seeds.

5. The Fast

• The extended fast can take seven to ten days or longer, up to even thirty days or longer. See pp. 119–29 for more information on extended fasting. Fasting is purifying—generally the most intense period of purification is in the first three days of a fast. Naturally, if one has prepared for the fast as described above, then the more difficult symptoms of purification will generally have already been passed through, and the transition to fasting can be relatively easeful.

It is very important to engage the period of preparation for fasting and not to jump directly into fasting (unless you are already very experienced at fasting and are already living a pure and balanced diet as a general life-habit). An easeful transition into fasting is assisted (for those who need it) with the liver flush (the night before the fast) and daily enemas (during the fast—generally in the morning before bathing). See the appendices that describe these practices.

6. Embracing the Searchless Raw Diet

• When it is time to break the fast, begin with whole (fruit or vegetable) juices instead of the diluted juices of the fast. This phase may be satisfying and last for many days. However, generally one is soon ready to recommence eating, now on the totally raw diet. This diet is principally based on greens, with added fruits, seeds, and some nuts as required. Re-introduce the blended green drinks and build again to 1–2 quarts (1–2 liters) a day, remembering to vary the greens regularly.

7. Ongoing Dietary and Fasting Approach

• Having now transitioned to the searchless raw diet, you will naturally choose to cycle between the fasting (purifying) phase and the nutritive phase of right diet, as Avatar Adi Da has described. This may be done simply by missing a meal, taking only liquid meals or juices for a day or more, or fasting one day per week. You may also intentionally re-engage an extended fast one (or more) times per year. All such decisions are based on sensitivity to the body—its general well-being, its inherent energy, eliminative symptoms, congestion, organ strength, or (when possible) based on monitoring the body directly, via blood pressure, blood sugar levels, the Chinese pulses, weight, urine pH levels, and/or other measures.

Alternative Dietary Transitions

Depending on the inherent strength of the body and other factors, some may not be able to transition to the raw diet using the extended fast. If this is the case, first engage the dietary transitions as described above, to the point of eliminating animal products. Simultaneous with dietary adaptation, develop sensitivity to the etheric being (or field of personal life-energy) through "conscious exercise", which integrates the gross body, the energy body, and the mind through the exercise of breath and feeling as well as specific physical exercises. Without the development of this etheric sensitivity, the energetic qualities of food will remain mysterious and diet will be managed mechanically rather than consciously. Without etheric sensitivity, a raw diet will tend to lead to excessive loss of weight, distress and cravings, and exaggerated symptoms of purification.

Here are two suggested methods of transition to the searchless raw diet for those who cannot engage an extended fast:

1. Systematic Elimination of Cooked Foods

It may be useful to engage the elimination of cooked foods gradually, in the following progression:

- bread and cooked grains (except rice)
- cooked vegetables (except potato)
- potato and rice

2. Gradual Elimination of Cooked Meals

It may be found that it is useful to eliminate cooked foods by maintaining occasional cooked meals and gradually eliminating the cooked foods. This could be done in one of the following ways:

- Eat two raw meals a day for a while before converting the third meal to raw food.

- Have exclusively raw meals one day a week for a while, increasing gradually to two days a week, and so forth. The transition to the totally raw diet will thus occur within six to seven weeks.

Managing Symptoms of Purification

Right dietary management is not common in the modern world. Thus, anyone who begins to conform to principles of right diet will likely experience some symptoms of purification. To consciously allow symptoms to arise and to know how to increase or decrease their intensity is the key to smooth passage through these transitions. Each person must discover through experimentation the ability to tolerate and properly manage these phenomena in order to lay the foundation for right dietary practice.

Many people have observed symptoms—such as headaches, dizziness, or inability to concentrate—after skipping a meal or just eating very lightly. Such symptoms are commonly interpreted in a negative way as signs of ill health, danger to the body, or incapacity to make necessary dietary changes. People feel, "I couldn't possibly eat that way forever—I'd get sick and perhaps even starve to death!"

However, such symptoms are generally and more rightly seen as evidence of a natural bodily process: When food intake decreases, a change occurs in the processes of metabolism that allows the body to eliminate accumulated wastes. As these toxic materials enter the bloodstream on their way to excretion, a great variety of symptoms can occur. For example:

- sensations of hunger or abdominal cramping
- muscle tensions and aches
- coated tongue, foul breath
- weakness and chronic fatigue
- dizziness and lightheadedness
- extreme bodily coldness or heat
- exaggerated emotions
- disturbed or restless sleep and disturbing dreams
- head and chest congestion, colds
- headache
- irritability
- rashes, boils
- inability to concentrate, light-headed feeling
- food cravings

If you react to these symptoms and eat a heavier (or more toxic) food immediately, they may go away—but you will have missed the opportunity for bodily purification.

On the other hand, eliminating a very toxic condition too rapidly (or severely) can render a person unable to function or susceptible to imbalance and possibly even a serious illness. Thus, embrace a form of gradual adaptation as described above—and also use common sense. If symptoms appear that seem out of proportion to the dietary change or if the symptoms continue for an undue period (for you), seek the advice of a properly trained physician—ideally one familiar with the theory and practice of the approach to health recommended by Avatar Adi Da Samraj.

It is always necessary to make responsible and intelligent adjustments as called for by any situation or sign in the body. For example, you might choose to increase or decrease the amount of blended green drinks you consume, decrease sweet fruits or use just non-sweet fruits, or even no fruits at all. If medically advised (and, generally, rarely), you may step back from the raw diet for a week or more by adding some brown rice or baked potato once or twice daily. If managed intelligently in this way, symptoms can be minimized while the process of purification continues and bodily energy and mental clarity increase.

3.
Foods for the Searchless Raw Diet

This section gives a basic indication of foods that are eaten on the searchless raw diet. Certain items listed may, of course, not be appropriate for a particular individual based on personal requirements (such as allergic reactions to certain types of food). And some of the foods listed are to be taken either in minimal amounts or in moderation. This is not intended to be a complete list, but, rather, a list of common examples to help you make choices, depending on locale and time of the year.

His Divine Presence Ruchira Avatar Adi Da Samraj has characterized the searchless raw diet as consisting principally of vegetables (primarily greens) and fruits, with some seeds and nuts.

NOTE: All raw, living foods should be taken in the most natural and healthful form possible. In other words, it is optimum if they are local (or, if imported, not adulterated in travel), pesticide-free, grown in a sustainable manner, not genetically modified or irradiated, and entirely non-toxic. Such food is more nutritious and generally tastes better than other foods, as well as being free from harmful substances. In *Green Gorilla*, and generally in Avatar Adi Da's dietary Instruction, the word "organic" is not used to define such quality, pure foods—because the word "organic" is associated with legal definitions that shift with time, locale, and economic realities.

Foods That Are Eaten

• **Greens (green leafy vegetables, wild edible greens, fresh herbs, sprouts, and grasses)**: These are especially to be taken in the form of blended green drinks, which are, in their most basic form, a combination of greens, fruit (to make the greens palatable), and water, mixed in a blender (which enables the nutrients of the greens to become easily assimilated, while maintaining the benefits of food roughage). This category includes "grasses"—such as wheatgrass, barley grass, etc.—either as whole blades in the blended green drink or in juice form.

• **Fruits**: This category is composed of sweet fruits (including bananas, dates, apples, papayas, pears, grapefruits, kiwis, pineapples, strawberries, and others) as well as "vegetable fruits" (which are non-sweet fruits that include tomatoes, cucumber, avocados, zucchini and other squashes, bell peppers, and others).

• **Leafy vegetables** (such as salad greens) **and flowers, pod vegetables** (typically legumes, in sprouted form), **stem vegetables** (such as celery, asparagus, etc.), **and root vegetables** (such as carrot, radish, jicama, daikon, ginger, etc). Note that pungent bulb vegetables (such as garlic, onions, and leeks) are not recommended, because they have been shown to impede communication between the two hemispheres of the brain. Also, tuberous root vegetables (such as potatoes, sweet potatoes, and yams) are generally not recommended for the raw diet, with the possible exception of chips made from dehydrated yams.

• **Seeds and nuts**, used sparingly. (For optimum digestion, seeds and nuts should be soaked overnight, or soaked and sprouted. Raw seed butter or raw nut butter would be used very sparingly, if at all.)

• **Sprouted seeds, nuts, and** (if agreeable to the individual's digestion) **sprouted legumes and grains**

• **Seaweeds** (such as nori, dulse, hijiki, kombu, arame)—washed and sun-dried, rather than boiled/cooked or dried at temperatures above 105° F (40.5° C)

• **Algae** (such as spirulina, chlorella, blue-green algae, etc.)

• **Fermented foods** (such as raw sauerkraut)

• **Other dehydrated foods** (such as raw crackers, dehydrated vegetable chips, etc.), in moderate amounts

• **Dried fruits** (in <u>small</u> <u>amounts</u>): preferably sun-dried, or dehydrated at a temperature below 105° F (40.5° C). As much as possible, dried fruit should be soaked before eating.

• **Possibly other raw foods** such as cacao (pure raw chocolate—beans, nibs, or powder) or maca

• **Herbal teas** (non-stimulating varieties, such as chamomile, peppermint, etc.)

> A note regarding water: Avatar Adi Da's recommendation is to use pure water that has been energized by exposure to sunlight, and stored in glass containers.

• **Sweeteners**: Acceptable natural sweeteners for minimal use include: raw agave or yacon nectar; stevia extract; pure xylitose; and potentially raw unfiltered honey. Dishes for the occasional celebratory meal can also be sweetened with dried figs, dates, raisins, etc.

Items not generally included in the searchless raw diet:

• **Salt**: Generally salt would not be used in the searchless raw diet. Minerals are already plentiful in the drinks and meals, and the natural flavors of the foods are attractive. If needed, then use minimal amounts of mineralized salt (such as Celtic Salt, Himalayan Crystal Salt, Real Salt—not iodized table salt), preferably directly to the tongue rather than mixed in with the food. Powdered dulse is a good salt substitute. Powdered kelp is also good.

• **Oils**: Oils are generally obtained directly from seeds or nuts or other elements in the diet. Added oils as a general rule would not be used, or, at most, small amounts of high quality, fresh (that is, not rancid), and un-heated vegetable oils (such as "extra virgin", expeller-pressed olive oil) may be usable (although not necessarily recommended) in salad dressings or as an ingredient in raw food dishes.

• **Caffeine-stimulants**: When a caffeine-containing stimulant is truly required, for functional or medicinal reasons, use green, white, or pu-erh teas. Avoid oolong or black teas. Coffee should be used only in the case of unavoidable necessity.

Foods for the Searchless Raw Diet

Primary foods

- **Greens**—primarily in blended drinks. Recommendation is 1–2 quarts (1–2 liters) of green drink per day. Green drinks may be taken as a meal on their own, or along with a fruit or vegetable meal (depending on what food combining works for the individual).

- **Fruits**—these would be included in the green drinks (for taste), and then could also be used in the context of a fruit-based meal. Seeds can also be taken with a fruit-based meal. In general, nuts (fats) do not combine well with fruit. (Such combinations are, once again, dependent on the individual case.)

Secondary foods

- **Vegetables**—can be taken in the context of a vegetable meal. Nuts or seeds can be taken with the vegetable meal.

- **Nuts and seeds**—in moderate amounts. For seeds, perhaps a cupped handful per day; for nuts, perhaps ten or so (for instance, ten almonds) a day.

- **Other foods on the "Foods That Are Eaten"** list on the preceding pages (pp. 105–106).

Foods Not Part of the Searchless Raw Diet

- Any form of cooked food

- Flesh foods (meat, poultry, fish) and eggs

- Milk and milk products

- Refined sugars (white sugar, brown sugar, corn syrup, maple syrup, etc.)

- Coffee (to be used only in the case of unavoidable necessity. See note on p. 107.)

- Flour

- Vinegar (lemon juice or lime juice are good alternatives)

- "Junk food" and "fast food"

- Chemical preservatives

- Refined or processed foods

- Genetically altered food (for example, GMO foods)

- Black or white pepper

- Mustard

- Gelatin

- Baking soda or powder

Sensitivity to the Body's Need
for Introducing Additional Foods

In the course of practicing the searchless raw dietary approach, it is rare but possible that—based on right and knowledgeable medical supervision and accountability—there may be cases when the body needs foods not normally on the raw diet, and/or cooked foods (possibly including animal protein). In His Instructions on the searchless raw diet, Avatar Adi Da has communicated the importance of observing the body's signs and seeing when and where it is displaying resistances to the simple raw regime. These resistances may particularly be observed by those in the early adaptation phases to the searchless raw diet, by those who are overenthusiastic or misinformed about the purification element of the raw diet, and by those in later stages of terminal illnesses (or other conditions where the inherent energy of the body is depleted or critically low)—especially if these individuals are new to the raw diet. In these and other situations, it is important to be sensitive to the right and lawful reasons for making use of less purifying foods. Avatar Adi Da admonishes His devotees to discuss this with a representative of the Radiant Life Clinic, or another qualified health practitioner who is sympathetic with the raw dietary approach Given by Avatar Adi Da Samraj. Such consultation is extremely useful, because independent decisions are often made on the basis of entrenched and generally uninspected habits and eating patterns, as well as various addictions and misinformation.

4.
Basic Guidelines for the Searchless Raw Diet

• Foods eaten are all raw (from among the raw foods listed in the previous section).

• Do not eat foods that toxify and enervate you, or lead to imbalances.

• Systematically undereat, as overeating taxes the body's mechanisms. However, this is not to encourage undernourishing, or to idealize skinniness. Eat enough food so that you are adequately nourished and do not feel starved (this amount varies from person to person and may vary for any individual from time to time). Obviously, optimum weight is a good indicator as well—so be aware of the range that is appropriate for your height, as well as being aware that those on a raw diet may have a lower optimum weight range than those who eat a more conventional diet.

• Do not eat foods to which you react.

• Take liquids moderately, if at all, during meals (other than green drinks).

• Chew your food thoroughly, and eat only to the point of being moderately full.

• Eat happily, free of reactive moods, and free from stress or the sense of having to hurry.

• Adapt to the dietary discipline described by Avatar Adi Da, but avoid "lunch-righteousness" (the tendency to make overmuch of the diet by being self-righteous about your own dietary purity, and overly critical of the dietary "errors" of others).

• Observe the effects of different food combinations on your particular constitution and regulate your diet accordingly. (You may find it useful to refer to literature on food combining.)

• Stay hydrated: Drink water throughout the day, as necessary (given that you take a lot of fluids already with the blended green drinks).

• Study Avatar Adi Da's Word on dietary practice, and also study the other recommended literature on raw diet. (See "For Further Study", pp. 130–134.)

• Intensify practice of "conscious exercise" and "conductivity". (See glossary.)

• Practice food-taking as a "conductivity" practice of conscious reception and release.

• Avoid the use of aluminum utensils and containers that contain Bisphenol-A (BPA)* as these can cause toxicity in food.

• The diet should be optimally healthful, serving energy and attention for practice of the process of Realization. This, rather than the sheer attractiveness of the food, is the primary principle (although right diet should also basically taste good and be attractive and pleasingly presented).

• In general, simpler is better, and, over time, will be preferred. Complicated "cuisine-y" or "raw gourmet" dishes would generally not be used, except, perhaps, on special celebratory occasions.

---

* Bisphenol-A (BPA) is an organic compound that is often used in the manufacture of clear plastic bottles and the lining of food and beverage containers. Long-term low-dose exposure to BPA is thought to induce chronic toxicity and hormonal imbalances in the human body.

• Bodily, emotional, and mental signs should be observed and taken into account in your process of dietary adaptation (keeping in mind that there may very well be some uncomfortable purification involved—which does not necessarily mean that your current diet is wrong for you).

• The diet should be one you can sustain, meaning that it can be lived as your ongoing approach to diet. There are a number of factors involved in this: education in right dietary principles, observing your bodily responses to different elements of the diet and adjusting appropriately, right consultation on the diet, not overdoing fats or sweets, using enough of the blended green drinks, and being accountable to others as you make adjustments to the diet.

5.
Preparing Blended Green Drinks

To make about 32 oz. (1 quart/1 liter) of blended green drink:

• Use a blender that is as powerful as you can obtain. It is generally optimum to have a 2–4 hp blender, such as a Vita-Mix or other high-powered blender.

• Rinse the ingredients before placing them in the blender.

• Start with 16 oz. (2 cups/475 ml) of one or more varieties of green leafy vegetable—such as kale, chard, collard greens, spinach, romaine lettuce, bok choy, arugula, etc.

You may also wish to add edible weeds (such as dandelion, lambsquarters, plantain, etc.), herbs (dill, basil, cilantro, mint, parsley, etc.), sprouts (alfalfa, clover, buckwheat, sunflower, etc.), other vegetables (celery, cucumber, etc.), or medicinal plants (such as aloe vera).

• Add small amounts of one or more fruits (to taste) to make the blended greens more palatable—such as apple, pineapple, banana, papaya, mango, pear, lemon, berries, and so on. When you begin making blended green drinks, experiment with the amount of fruit. The general recommendation is to use less fruits than greens, but you may want to use somewhat more fruit than greens at first, and then over time use less so that you develop a "greener" drink.

It is also possible to make blended green drinks using greens with non-sweet fruit vegetables (such as tomatoes, cucumber, zucchini and other squashes, bell peppers, etc.), or other vegetables, sprouts, etc., rather than with sweet fruits—and, for some, this may be necessary because of their bodily reaction to sweet fruits.

Further healthful additions to the basic green drink recipe are also possible, such as a spoonful of ground flax-seed, some chlorella, spirulina, or blue-green algae, or wheatgrass juice, a bit of lemon juice or lime juice, etc.

• Add 16 oz. (2 cups/475 ml) of pure water.

• Blend well. It takes generally about thirty seconds for a high-powered blender. With a lower-powered bender, you may have to blend longer—but do not blend for so long that you heat the drink (or overheat the blender).

• Drink as much as you want/need immediately. Any extra can be stored in the refrigerator for eight hours easily, and even up to seventy-two hours.

NOTE: It is important to rotate the greens regularly, to avoid micro-accumulation of alkaloids contained in a single variety of greens, which may over time create toxicity in the body. Use as wide a variety of greens as possible.*

---

* See Victoria Boutenko's book *Green for Life* for more information on this point.

6.
Sample Meal Plan

The following is a <u>sample</u> daily meal plan for the searchless raw diet, intended <u>only</u> as a platform for individuals to experiment in finding their own minimum-optimum cycle of meal-taking (accounting for your own discoveries about optimum food-combining and types/amounts of food to consume, and the optimum balance of fruit and vegetable meals that works for you). Keep in mind that the meals should, generally, be simple and straightforward, rather than being a kind of "raw cuisine", and that fats should be kept to an appropriate level while making sure that you are not undernourishing yourself and that food-taking is an essentially pleasing experience.

BREAKFAST (between 7 a.m. and 8 a.m.)

Blended green drink (10–16 oz. [1¼–2 cups/300–475 ml], or more)—usually taken before eating any solid food

and possibly:

a fruit meal and seeds

LUNCH (between 12 p.m. and 1 p.m.)

Blended green drink (10–16 oz. [1¼–2 cups/300–475 ml], or more)—usually taken before eating solid food

followed by either:

Fruit meal consisting of one or more fruits of the same kind or of different varieties, and maybe some seeds. For example, one could use one or more (or all) of these suggestions:

- A plate of sliced apple and pear, with a dip made of pureed kiwi fruit
- A bowl of berries
- A plate of tropical fruit slices—such as papaya and pineapple
- A small plate of citrus fruits (as long as you do not have problems combining citrus with other fruits)
- A small amount of seeds—for example, about a cupped handful of sunflower seeds (preferably soaked for twelve hours) and a tablespoon (15 ml) of ground flaxseed

or:

Vegetable meal consisting of greens, non-sweet fruits (such as tomatoes, cucumber, avocados, zucchini and other squashes, bell peppers, etc.), seaweeds, sprouts, simple dips and dressings, raw crackers, and maybe some nuts and/or seeds. For example, one could use one or more (or all) of these suggestions:

- A large green salad
- Various sprouts, possibly wrapped in raw nori
- Sticks of non-sweet fruits and other vegetables, including root vegetables, with a dip of blended red pepper
- Raw seed crackers
- A small amount of nuts, for example, ten almonds
- Ground flaxseed

DINNER (between 6 p.m. and 8 p.m.)

Blended green drink (10–16 oz. [1¼–2 cups/300–475 ml] —usually taken before eating solid food

followed by:

the alternate meal to the one taken at lunch

R aw recipe books often give the impression that they are making a concession to people who are actually craving to maintain old dietary habits, and who are not really understanding the raw-diet approach, which involves the body distinguishing between the different foods it takes in the context of a natural, wild circumstance.

Non-humans chew things one at a time. They know what they are having each time they eat. They do not send a bunch of ingredients to the chef to make something not otherwise identifiable.

The body depends on being able to differentiate between the different foods it takes, because each food has different chemical characteristics. The body also distinguishes color and other qualities of how a food looks, as well as taste, aroma, freshness, and so on. The body wants to make that discriminative address to everything it takes as food—and foods also taste better when they are eaten "straight".

"Raw cuisine" does not permit such direct address. Raw diet recipe books often try to make cuisine out of raw food, to make some kind of "event" or "entertainment" out of raw food—to make it more or less addictive. Such things are all right sometimes, when you have a special occasion—but, generally, day to day, the ability to discriminate each food is a basic principle to uphold.

—His Divine Presence
Ruchira Avatar Adi Da Samraj

7.
A Brief Guide to Fasting

Avatar Adi Da recommends periodic fasting as an essential element of the searchless raw dietary approach:

As a basic means to quicken the effectiveness of your by-Me-Given (and formally expected) obligation to constantly and intensively maintain the "self"-discipline of bodily purification, bodily rebalancing, and bodily rejuvenation (or bodily regeneration), your dietary practice should also include right occasional and periodic fasting (unless you are otherwise rightly medically advised). Therefore, unless your bodily state (of fully achieved purification) and the purity of your daily food-intake do not (at any present moment) require it, your dietary practice should (in the general case) also (as necessary) include appropriate occasional (twenty-four-hour, or longer) and regular (extended) periodic fasting. Long fasts are (in the general case) to be engaged periodically or at least once per year (unless right medical advice prohibits such, or, otherwise, an exceptional state of bodily and dietary purity makes such, at any present moment, unnecessary)—and, to be effective, they should be continued for at least seven to ten days, and up to three or four weeks (or even longer). In addition, shorter or longer periods of totally raw mono-diet may also be engaged for the purpose of continuing the process of bodily purification during periods of time before and after fasting—but such temporary (rather than regular and constant) raw-mono-diet exercises should (in the general case) be engaged only in addition to fasting, and not as an alternative to fasting.

—His Divine Presence
Ruchira Avatar Adi Da Samraj
(pp. 36–37)

Basic Fasting Guidelines

Decide on your fasting plan, in discussion with a licensed medical practitioner (optimally, a member of the Radiant Life Clinic, versed in Avatar Adi Da's approach to diet). If you have not fasted before, or if you have had difficulty fasting in the past, it is especially important to talk to a licensed medical practitioner. (If you are taking drugs under a doctor's care, even naturopathic remedies, be sure to consult your doctor before planning and preparing for a fast.)

Preparing for a Fast

• Begin your fasting/diet diary, recording what you consume and when, and the effects you experience bodily, emotionally, mentally, and in your total life-practice.

• Gradually simplify your diet, eating only raw fruits and vegetables (no nuts, seeds, or vitamins or other supplements) for the period before beginning the fast. You should not stop forms of hormone replacement therapy unless under medical supervision. (See also the note about medications, pp. 96–97 in "Intelligent Dietary Transitions".)

• Especially if you are planning an intense form of fasting such as the lemon-water fast, it is useful to do significant preliminary purification: as much as a week on the raw diet and possibly a liver flush.

• Remember that there are no hard and fast rules for fasting, breaking the fast, etc. It is always a matter of feeling and observing your personal experience.

During the Fast

• If you are not experienced with lemon-water fasts, we suggest that for the first three days of the fast you use fruit juice (strained and diluted with water—at least 50 percent). Take perhaps 8 oz. (240 ml) or so every two to four hours, or else 8–16 oz. (240–475 ml) of diluted juice at mealtimes. (Be sure to also drink plenty of water in between your juice consumption! And strain your juices well to eliminate pulp, which can activate the digestive system and cause hunger.)

• Then, for the most intense purification, go on the lemon-water fast, using water and lemon juice (approximately one part lemon juice to nine or ten parts water) without sweetener. Continue with your water consumption. (Drink a minimum of 64 oz. [2 quarts/2 liters] of liquid a day.)

• If you have a condition of particularly low blood sugar, you can remedy this by taking a small amount of diluted (50 percent) fruit juice a few times during the day while you are fasting on lemon water, or possibly adding a small amount of agave or some other appropriate raw sweetener to your lemon water (1 tbsp. [15 ml] per 10 oz. [300 ml] of water/ lemon mixture).

• De-emphasize worldly entertainments and abstain from sexual activity; emphasize devotional practices; study; intensify the practice of "conductivity" and "conscious exercise".

• Make use of enemas or other forms of bowel irrigation as needed (the recommendation for the first days of the fast is once a day, in the morning). The use of enemas is most helpful during the first few days of fasting—some fasters find bowel irrigation unnecessary later on in the fast (and some fasting experts don't use it at all). See appendix B.

• If you are concerned about weight loss or other symptoms, consult a licensed medical practitioner who is qualified to identify signs when the fast should stop for health reasons.

• If you are experiencing significant symptoms of purification such as lightheadedness, tiredness, dizziness, etc., be cautious about driving, operating heavy machinery, etc. (These symptoms may be significantly minimized by right preparation for a fast, and by drinking sufficient amounts of water throughout the fast, and they may also be lessened through daily bowel hygiene/enemas.) Be intelligent, responsible, and don't do anything that could be hazardous to yourself or others.

• Optimally, you would continue the fast until the basic cleansing is complete—as shown by signs such as weight stabilization (or only slow weight loss), and the return of hunger. (The health representative supervising your fast will help you determine when this point is reached. The basic cleansing will not necessarily occur within the seven to ten day period, so you may need to decide whether or not to continue or end the fast before the cleansing is complete. Check with your health representative.) Then start to add fruit juices (starting with, perhaps, three 8 oz. [240 ml] glasses of undiluted juice per day, or six 8 oz. [240 ml] glasses of diluted juice) and then, perhaps, vegetable juices and/or "de la Torre" drink (recipe is given in appendix D). (Determine what you consume by what you feel attracted to—smell, taste, appearance, etc. If you are attracted to them, tropical fruit juices, such as pineapple or papaya, or else prune juice, may be good for helping digestion start.)

• You may stay on this "juice diet" as long as the body has high energy and you are enjoying a sense of bodily well-being.

Breaking the Fast

• Transition back to solid food slowly. Take approximately one day of transition for every three days of fasting.

• Begin the first day with two or three small meals, taking raw fruit only—perhaps half an apple, or 4 oz. ($^1/_2$ cup/15g) of pineapple, or 4 oz. ($^1/_2$ cup/15g) of grapes at each meal. (Make your choice based on what you feel attracted to.) The second day, increase your intake a bit. Eat slowly and chew well. Maintain your feeling-sensitivity, and evaluate how the food you take affects your overall energy and your free attention. This process of gradual adaptation to solid food may take a number of days. If you have been using enemas or other forms of bowel irrigation, discontinue them when you start eating solid food.

• Eat in an attractive, calm, nurturing environment, and in a relaxed manner.

• Continue to drink significant amounts of water, a suggested amount being eight 8 oz. [240 ml] glasses of water and/or juice per day.

• During this period, bowel functioning should start again (signs that bowel function has resumed include hunger, a gurgling stomach and, finally, defecation). If there are no signs of digestion (gurgling, etc.) occurring after the second day of the process of adaptation to solid food, check with an appropriately qualified licensed medical practitioner. Tropical fruits such as pineapple and papaya, or soaked prunes, may be helpful in getting your digestive process moving. You may also find it helpful to use powdered psyllium seed husks, thoroughly mixed with water, to help move things through.

• On the first day of transitioning back to solid food, reintroduce the blended green drinks, beginning with 16 oz. (2 cups/475 ml) then 32 oz. (1 quart/1 liter), then more (48–64 oz. [6–8 cups/1.5–2 liters]) on consecutive days.

• Gradually introduce more items into your diet, as seems necessary and useful—first, raw fruits and vegetables, and, then, if desired, raw seeds and nuts. This is an important transition, during which the body goes through changes, just as it did during the fast.

• Order of introducing foods after the fast/liquid diet:

  • blended green drinks

  • juicy fruits (citrus fruits, apples, etc.)

  • fruit vegetables (tomatoes, cucumber, etc.)

  • starchy fruits such as bananas

  • sprouts

  • other raw vegetables (non-fruit type) that can be eaten raw such as carrots, celery, etc. (Most authorities agree that vegetables like potatoes and sweet potatoes should not be eaten raw.)

  • seeds and nuts, used sparingly (for optimum digestion, these should be soaked, or soaked and sprouted)

  • oily fruits such as avocados

  • then, the whole range of foods that can be eaten on the fully raw diet (seaweeds, etc.)

Returning to Right Dietary Practice

• Let the body feel into what it needs and wants.

• Use the sense of smell to guide what type of food you choose, and how much you eat.

• Eat food that is entirely non-toxic (as described previously).

• If possible, it is preferable to eat food that is harvested when ripe.

• Study the recommended books in "For Further Study", pp. 130–34.

• Experiment with your diet to see if any variations are useful or necessary.

• Adjust your diet based on your feeling-sensitivity to what is going on in the body-mind. Signs of toxicity in the body-mind might indicate that you should be on a more eliminative diet (fasting) for a time. Signs of depletion might indicate the need for a more nutrient-rich diet for a time (increased green drinks, etc.).

Brief Summary of the Lemon-Water Fast

Protocol of approach for an extended cleansing fast (recommended to be engaged, as a general rule, once or more per year):

1. Engage this fast for seven to ten days (or longer, with appropriate medical consultation).

2. Basic fast: lemon juice and water (one part lemon to nine parts water)
   - Minimum 64 oz. (2 quarts/2 liters) per day (some can be water alone)
   - Use of other juices based on medical recommendation only
   - For hypoglycemia symptoms (weakness, dizzyness, loss of mental sharpness), treat with one or two 8 oz. (240 ml) glasses of diluted fruit juice per day until the symptoms are controlled (usually one 8 oz. [240 ml] glass is sufficient)
   - If weight loss is too rapid, and/or weakness is experienced:

     A) Check for sufficient fluids (minimum 64 oz. [2 quarts/2 liters] per day)

     B) Add one or more 8 oz. (240 ml) glasses of diluted juices

   - Beyond the cleansing point (when weight is stabilized, meaning only slow weight loss is occurring; when hunger is restored), then, begin a juice diet. First begin to add fruit juices then vegetable juices.

3. Continue with the transition back to solid food.

Who Should Fast, and When

For some people, fasting is inappropriate. Here are some guidelines from the Radiant Life Clinic based on our own experimentation and our consideration of the research of others. If you have a question, consult with a licensed medical practitioner (optimally, a member of the Radiant Life Clinic).

You <u>should</u> <u>not</u> fast if:

• You are pregnant or nursing a child.

• You are under the age of fifteen (unless specifically approved to fast and monitored by a qualified health practitioner).

If you fall into any of the following categories, *check with an appropriately qualified licensed medical practitioner* before fasting:

• You have a chronic or debilitating illness that is also an enervating health problem, with insufficient inherent bodily strength to fast.

• You lose weight excessively and rapidly during a fast, out of all proportion to your body size, and you have difficulty regaining it. (During the fast, it is important to maintain fluid intake, bowel hygiene, exercise, and "conductivity" practice. In other words, it is important to breathe and maintain the feeling of vitality and strength in the energy core of the body—the navel region—and not to succumb to vital weakness or "spaciness".)

• You are currently or have recently been using any drugs (prescription or non-prescription). This situation requires medical consultation and direct monitoring.

• You suffer from emaciation. Those suffering from emaciation should only fast under the direct supervision of a naturally-oriented medical doctor. At most, short fasts interspersed with a raw diet (emphasizing protein-rich green vegetables) or a diet that may include cooked food (when medically advised) that builds energy and muscle would be recommended until full energy and weight have been restored.

• You suffer from significant mental or emotional illness.

Most people can fast healthfully. Check with an appropriately qualified licensed medical practitioner before deciding <u>not</u> to fast!

Mono-Diet

Those for whom it is not advisable to fast may benefit from a fruit "mono-diet"—eating one kind of fruit exclusively for several days. (Note: Be sure the food you choose is not one to which you are allergic.)

The fruit should be raw and fresh. Almost any fruit may be taken on a mono diet, except those with a high concentration of carbohydrates, such as bananas. Grapes and apples are the most benign and purifying for the body (though some people may find apples difficult to digest, in which case grapes should be used). These fruits allow the body to maintain a high level of energy and, at the same time, to purify itself of toxins and to shed excess weight.

Because of their high sugar content, limit the quantity of grapes you take to 32–48 oz. (2–3 lbs./1–1.4 kg) per day. Eat only ripe grapes. Some authorities recommend that you also consume all of the seeds and skins to aid digestion and elimination.

Citrus fruits and citrus juices cause toxins in the body to be released very quickly. Therefore, they are generally best used in combination with other fruits and fruit juices, rather than exclusively, and are generally not a good choice for a mono-diet.

If you want to sustain the mono-diet for longer than a day or two, apply the principles for preparing for, sustaining, and breaking a fast given on pp. 120–25.

8.
For Further Study

Titles from "The Epitome of Seventh-Stage and Traditional Esotericism" bibliographical list, compiled by His Divine Presence Ruchira Avatar Adi Da Samraj:

The Yoga of Right Diet: An Intelligent Approach To Dietary Practice That Supports Communion With The Living Divine Reality, by the Avataric Great Sage, Adi Da Samraj. Middletown, Calif.: The Dawn Horse Press, 2006.

Raw Gorilla: The Principles of Regenerative Raw Diet Applied In True Spiritual Practice—As Lived By Members of the Johannine Daist Communion Under The Guidance of the Divine Adept Da Free John [Adi Da Samraj]. Prepared by the Radiant Life Clinic and Research Center Based on the Wisdom-Teaching of Da Free John [Adi Da Samraj]. Clearlake, Calif.: The Dawn Horse Press, 1982.

The Eating Gorilla Comes In Peace: The Transcendental Principle of Life Applied To Diet and The Regenerative Discipline of True Health, by Heart-Master Da Love-Ananda [Adi Da Samraj]. San Rafael, Calif.: The Dawn Horse Press, 1979.

The China Study: The Most Comprehensive Study of Nutrition Ever Conducted and the Startling Implications for Diet, Weight Loss, and Long-Term Health, by T. Colin Campbell and Thomas M. Campbell II. Dallas: Benbella Books, 2006.

In Defense of Food: An Eater's Manifesto, by Michael Pollan. New York: Penguin Press, 2008.

The History of Natural Hygiene: The Basic Teachings of Doctors Jennings, Graham, Trall, and Tilden, by Hereward Carrington, and *Principles of Natural Hygiene*, by Herbert M. Shelton. Mokelumne Hill, Calif.: Health Research, 2nd ed., 1964.

"The Epitome of Seventh-Stage and Traditional Esotericism"

Avatar Adi Da Samraj has created a library collection and associated bibliography (interspersed with His commentary) of many thousands of books, articles, and audio-visual materials, each item selected from the many more thousands of items on aspects of the Great Tradition He has reviewed over the past several decades. This complete collection is entitled *The Basket of Tolerance*. "The Epitome of Seventh-Stage and Traditional Esotericism" is a smaller essential list (drawn from the larger collection), emphasizing the "esoteric" (or Spiritually and Transcendentally oriented) endeavors of humankind, including the foundation practices necessary for such endeavors (including right dietary practice). Thus, the books and articles listed on the Epitome of Seventh-Stage and Traditional Esotericism represent those which Avatar Adi Da regards as most useful to study on the full range of topics related to true esoteric teaching and practice. ■

Toxemia Explained, by J. H. Tilden, MD. Mokelumne Hill, Calif.: Health Research, 1968.

Fasting and Eating for Health: A Medical Doctor's Program for Conquering Disease, by Joel Fuhrman. New York: St. Martin's Griffin, 1995.

Short Cut: Regeneration Through Fasting, by Julia Seton. New York: Cosimo Classics, 2006.

Fasting Path: The Way to Spiritual, Physical, and Emotional Enlightenment, by Stephen Harrod Buhner. New York: Avery, 2003.

Fantastic Voyage: Live Long Enough to Live Forever, by Ray Kurzweil and Terry Grossman, MD. Emmaus, Penn.: Rodale, 2004.

"Harmony with Nature in Chinese Thought and Opposition to Nature in Western Thought", by Olof G. Lidin. Hirakata City, Osaka, Japan: Intercultural Research Institute, The Kansai University of Foreign Studies, 1974.

"Yin-Yang", by Robin R. Wang. *The Internet Encyclopedia of Philosophy*. www.iep.utm.edu (retrieved May 11, 2008)

"Yin and Yang Theory", pp. 7–15 in *The Web That Has No Weaver: Understanding Chinese Medicine*, by Ted J. Kaptchuk. New York: McGraw-Hill, 2000.

Anna Yoga: The Yoga of Food, by Jack Santa Maria. London: Rider, 1978.

The Yoga of Eating: The Role of Food in Self-Realization, by Satya Narayana Dasa and Gerda Staes. Vrindavana, Mathura, U.P., India: Jiva Institute, 2007.

Grain Damage: Rethinking the High-Starch Diet, by Douglas N. Graham. Key Largo, Fla.: Foodnsport Press, 2005.

"Why All Should Eat Only Raw Foods Always", by Dr. Bernarr. www.living-foods.com (retrieved April 15, 2008)

The Live Food Factor: A Comprehensive Guide to the Ultimate Diet for Body, Mind, Spirit, and Planet, by Susan Schenck. San Diego: Awakenings Publications, 2006.

Achieving Great Health, by Bob McCauley. Lansing, Mich.: Watershed Wellness Center, 2005.

Green Foods Bible: Everything You Need to Know About Barley Grass, Wheatgrass, Kamut, Chlorella, Spirulina and More, by David Sandoval. Topanga, Calif.: Freedom Press, 2007.

Rebuild Your Health with High Energy Enzyme Nourishment, by Ann Wigmore. Boston: Ann Wigmore Foundation, 1991.

The Hippocrates Diet and Health Program, by Ann Wigmore. With foreword by Dennis Weaver. Wayne, N.J.: Avery Publishing, 1984.

The Wheatgrass Book, by Ann Wigmore. Wayne, New Jersey: Avery Publishing, 1985.

Blending Book: Maximizing Nature's Nutrients: How to Blend Fruits and Vegetables for Better Health, by Ann Wigmore. New York: Avery, 1997.

Green for Life, by Victoria Boutenko. Ashland, Ore.: Raw Family Publishing, 2005.

"How My Family Eats", by Victoria Boutenko. *Raw Family Newsletter*, October 2006. www.rawfamily.com (retrieved April 5, 2008)

"February's Popular Green Smoothie Questions Answered by Victoria [Boutenko]". *Raw Family Newsletter*, February 2006. www.rawfamily.com (retrieved April 2, 2008)

"Seven Common Mistakes That Occur on Raw Foods", by Victoria Boutenko. *Raw Family Newsletter*, January 2007. www.rawfamily.com (retrieved April 3, 2008)

"One More Benefit of Practicing Gratitude: It Can Help You Stay Raw!", by Victoria Boutenko. *Raw Family Newsletter*, November 2006. www.rawfamily.com (retrieved April 9, 2008)

"Jaw Exercise", by Victoria Boutenko. *Raw Family Newsletter*, January 2006. www.rawfamily.com (retrieved April 3, 2008)

12 Steps to Raw Foods, by Victoria Boutenko. Ashland, Ore.: Raw Family, revised and expanded edition, 2007.

Quantum Eating: The Ultimate Elixir of Youth, by Tonya Zavasta. Cordova, Tenn.: BR Publishing, 2007.

"Gaining and Losing Weight the Quantum Way!", by Tonya Zavasta. *Beautiful on Raw Newsletter*, November 2007. www.beautifulonraw.com (retrieved April 2, 2008)

"Wild Greens and Health", by David Wolfe. www.thebestdayever.com (retrieved April 5, 2008)

The Sunfood Diet Success System: 36 Lessons in Health Transformation, by David Wolfe. San Diego, Calif.: Sunfood Publishing, 7th ed., 2008.

The 80/10/10 Diet, by Dr. Douglas N. Graham. Key Largo, Fla.: FoodnSport Press, 2006.

Sunfood Living: Resource Guide for Global Health, by John McCabe. Foreword by David Wolfe. Berkeley: North Atlantic Books, 2007.

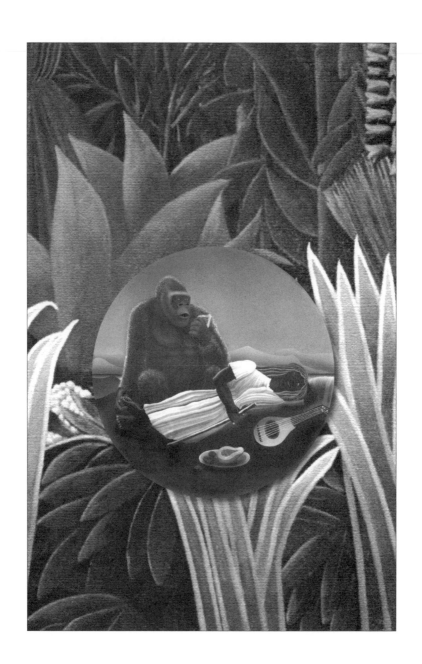

EPILOGUE

Right Principle and Right Self-Management: The Secrets of How To Change

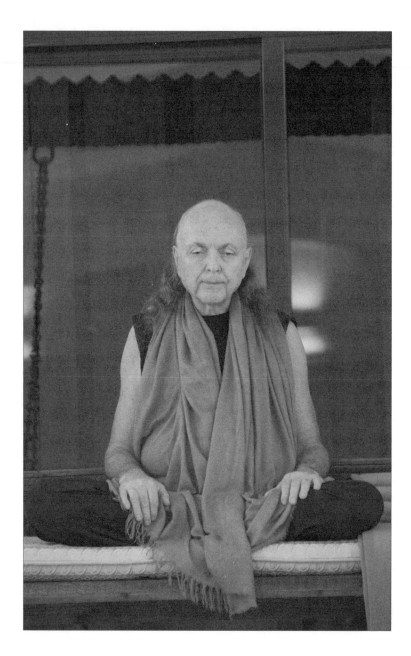

Right Principle and Right Self-Management: The Secrets of How To Change

An Essay by
His Divine Presence
Ruchira Avatar Adi Da Samraj

The following essay is part of Avatar Adi Da's principal text, The Aletheon, *in which He addresses His devotees about the secrets of living the practice of "right life" in relationship to Him. However, Avatar Adi Da's Wisdom can be useful to anyone in making any life-change.*

True and sustainable change and positive, mature human adaptation are not made on the basis of any "self"-conscious reaction-resistance to old, degenerative, and immature habits.

True and positive change is not a matter of <u>not</u> doing something.

True and positive change is always a matter of doing something <u>else</u>—something that is inherently right, free, pure and purifying, balanced and re-balancing, truly regenerative, and, altogether, a matter of functional equanimity.

True and positive change is always a matter of <u>both</u> right principle (based on right understanding, and, especially, right "self"-understanding) and right (and consistently applied) "self"-management.

Therefore, you must be intrinsically open and free to always feel and participate in modes of "self"-managing life-functioning that are new and right.

The habit-tendencies and habit-patterns of your casually accumulated life-adaptations are not wrong.

All your habit-tendencies and habit-patterns were appropriate enough in their own moment of first happening—and there is no need to feel guilt or despair about them.

All seeking-efforts to change your accumulated habit-tendencies and habit-patterns by strategically opposing them are basically and inevitably fruitless.

All seeking-efforts are forms of the dramatization of "self"-conflict, and, therefore, they only reinforce the habitual modes of ego-possession.

What is simply not used is intrinsically obsolete—whereas what is opposed is constantly kept in front of you.

The creative principle of true and positive change is a combination of always relaxed inspection (and discriminating awareness) of existing tendencies and, on that basis, an active, persistent, full feeling-orientation to right, new, and regenerative functional patterns.

If this creative principle of true and positive change is practiced consistently and in ecstatic (or intrinsically ego-transcending) resort to Me, the Divine Avataric Master, free growth—demonstrated as habit-transcending true and positive change—is assured.

Have no regrets.

Resort to Me moment to moment, and under all circumstances.

All that has been done by anyone had its logic in its time. Only I avail.

Whatever is your habit in this moment is not wrong—but it is simply a beginning.

No habit is necessary, because every habit is only a temporary and merely conditionally existing (and, thus, entirely changeable) pattern.

Every habit-pattern is merely <u>tending</u> to persist, because it has not yet been replaced by true and positive changes of pattern itself.

Always listen to Me, always resort to Me, always practice My "Radical" Reality-Teaching of Truth, and always understand and act in accordance with what is the right, free, and regenerative pattern of each psycho-physical life-function of the human being.

Always Stand Intrinsically Prior to all negative judgements about what you have done and what you tend to do.

Always intensively engage the happy ordeal of habit-transcending new adaptation in ecstatic devotional Communion with Me, the Divine Avataric Master.

I <u>Am</u> the Unbroken (Indivisible and Indestructible) Transcendental Spiritual and Self-Evidently Divine Conscious Light That "Lives" you.

I <u>Am</u> the Only One—Who <u>Is</u> Surrounding, Pervading, and <u>Being</u> you, and all, and All. ■

GLOSSARY

Adidam / Adidam Ruchiradam—When His Divine Presence Ruchira Avatar Adi Da Samraj spontaneously Gave the name "Adidam" (in January 1996) to the Reality-Way He has Revealed, He pointed out that the name "Adidam" evokes His Primal Self-Confession, "I Am Adi Da", or, more simply, "I Am Da".

"Ruchiradam" is a word newly coined by Avatar Adi Da, deriving from Sanskrit "Ruchira" (meaning "bright" or "radiant"). The compound reference "Adidam Ruchiradam" communicates that Adidam is the Way of devotion to Avatar Adi Da Samraj—Who Is the "Bright" Itself, and Who Gives the Realization of His own "Bright" Self-Condition. Furthermore, "Ruchira Dham Hermitage" is the name Avatar Adi Da gave to the place where He underwent a profound and unprecedented Yogic Event that marked the Perfection of His Revelation of the Reality-Way of Adidam. Thus, the name Adidam Ruchiradam honors that Event.

the "Bright"—With the phrase "the 'Bright'", Avatar Adi Da refers to the Self-Existing and Self-Radiant Divine Reality that He has Revealed since His Birth. Avatar Adi Da named His own Self-Evidently Divine Self-Condition "the 'Bright'" in His Infancy, as soon as He acquired the capability of language.

This term is placed in quotation marks to indicate that Avatar Adi Da uses it with the specific meaning described here.

"conductivity"—Avatar Adi Da's technical term for participation in (and responsibility for) the movement of natural bodily energies via intentional exercises of feeling and breathing. Such exercises include all of the right-life disciplines Given by Avatar Adi Da to His devotees—such as the searchless raw diet, meditation, "conscious exercise", emotional-sexual practices, sacramental worship, devotional service, etc. When Avatar Adi Da's devotee is Transcendentally-and-Spiritually awakened by Him, the devotee practices "Spirit-'conductivity'"—or participation in and responsibility for the movement of Avatar Adi Da's Divine Transcendental Spirit-Current of Love-Bliss in its natural course of association with the body-mind. (Avatar Adi Da's principal Instruction relative to the "general" or "basic" forms of Spirit-"conductivity" is Given in *The Dawn Horse Testament*.) The term "conductivity" is placed in quotation marks to indicate that Avatar Adi Da uses it with the specific technical meaning described here.

congregations of Adidam—In order to make it possible for all kinds of people to formally relate to Him, His Divine Presence Adi Da Samraj has created four "congregations" of the Reality-Way of Adidam. The congregations radiate like a mandala, or sacred pattern, from Avatar Adi Da at its heart.

• The **First Congregation** comprises those who engage the full and intensive process of "radical" devotion, right life, and "Perfect Knowledge" in the Reality-Way of Adidam—first as student-beginners, and then accepted into the Transcendental Spiritual process, and Awakening (ultimately) to Divine Self-Realization.

• The **Second Congregation** comprises the gathering of Avatar Adi Da's devotees who engage the foundational process of "radical" devotion and right life, and beginning "consideration" of Avatar Adi Da's essential "Perfect Knowledge" Teachings.

• The **Third Congregation** comprises the supportive gathering of those who respond to Avatar Adi Da Samraj and are moved to embrace a simple practice of "radical" devotion to Him and support of His Work. The third congregation also includes individuals who maintain a traditional religious affiliation, while also embracing the supportive obligations of this congregation.

• The **Fourth Congregation** comprises those from indigenous and traditional cultures around the world who devotionally respond to Avatar Adi Da Samraj and are moved to embrace a simple life of practice in relation to Him.

Beyond the congregations of Adidam stand many who respond to Avatar Adi Da, and choose to study or assist His Work without formally becoming His devotees. (See also **"radical" devotion, right life, and "Perfect Knowledge"**.)

"conscious exercise"—Avatar Adi Da's technical term for participation in and responsibility for the bodily and life-energy dimensions of existence via intentional exercises of feeling and breathing. "Conscious exercise" is the coordinated exercise of attention, feeling, breath, and body in association with the natural energy of the body-mind, and (in due course) with Avatar Adi Da's Spirit-Energy. "Conscious exercise" includes many practical disciplines of posture and breathing and specific exercise routines to be engaged as daily practices in the Reality-Way of Adidam—as indicated by Avatar Adi Da's definition of the term in *The Dawn Horse Testament*: "The Maintenance Of bodily Equanimity and physical Well-being Through Systematic Exercises and General bodily Practices That Conduct Natural human (and etheric) life-energy Throughout".

This term is placed in quotation marks to indicate that Avatar Adi Da uses it with the specific technical meaning described here.

devotional recognition-response—When the heart recognizes Avatar Adi Da as Reality Itself appearing in human form, there is inevitably the simultaneous impulse to devotionally respond to Him. The entire practice of the Reality-Way of Adidam is founded in this devotional heart-recognition of, and devotional heart-response to, Avatar Adi Da Samraj.

disciplines of the Reality-Way of Adidam (functional, practical, relational, and cultural)—The most basic functional, practical, and relational disciplines of the Reality-Way of Adidam are forms of appropriate human action and responsibility in relation to diet, health, exercise, sexuality, work, service to and support of Avatar Adi Da's Work, and cooperative association with other practitioners of the Reality-Way of Adidam. The most basic cultural obligations of the Reality-Way of Adidam include meditation, sacramental worship, study of Avatar Adi Da's Reality-Teaching (and also at least a basic discriminative study of the Great Tradition of religion and Spirituality that is the inheritance of humankind), and regular participation in the "form" (or schedule) of daily, weekly, monthly, and annual devotional activities and retreats. See also **"radical" devotion, right life, and "Perfect Knowledge"**.

ego-"I"—The presumption of separate and separative existence. The "I" is placed in quotation marks to indicate that it is used by Avatar Adi Da in the "so to speak" sense. He is communicating (by means of the quotation marks) that, in reality, there is no such thing as the separate "I", even though it appears to be the case from the "point of view" of ordinary human perception.

"emotional-sexual conscious exercise"—The preparatory sexual practice for Avatar Adi Da's Congregationist devotees, the basic elements of which are described in Avatar Adi Da's book *The Complete Yoga of Human Emotional-Sexual Life*. In the practice of "emotional-sexual conscious exercise", sexual activity is engaged in an intentionally relaxed manner that includes whole bodily participation, the bypassing of degenerative (and, in the male, ejaculatory) orgasm, and the regenerative "conductivity" of sexual energy. Avatar Adi Da Samraj describes the essence of "emotional-sexual conscious exercise" (and of all the Yogic emotional-sexual disciplines He has Given to His devotees) as "True Devotion To Me, Active Love Of one another, and Real (True and Mutual) Trust." (As practice matures, "emotional-sexual conscious exercise" becomes "emotional-sexual devotional Communion".)

"emotional-sexual devotional Communion"—The fully developed (and, Transcendentally Spiritually, fully technically responsible) sexual practice for Avatar Adi Da's Congregationist devotees (described in *The Dawn Horse Testament*). In the practice of "emotional-sexual devotional

Communion", sexual activity is fully engaged as a form of Transcendental Spiritual Divine Communion, and the tendency to degenerative orgasm is replaced by a regenerative pleasure that has positive effects in the body. As with "emotional-sexual conscious exercise", Avatar Adi Da Samraj describes the essence of "emotional-sexual devotional Communion" as "True Devotion To <u>Me</u>, <u>Active</u> Love Of one another, and Real (<u>True</u> and <u>Mutual</u>) Trust."

etheric—The etheric is the dimension of life-energy which functions through the human nervous system. The human body is surrounded and infused by this personal life-energy, felt as the play of emotions and life-force in the body.

Four Congregations of Adidam—see **congregations of Adidam**.

functional, practical, relational, and cultural disciplines—see **disciplines of the Reality-Way of Adidam (functional, practical, relational, and cultural)**.

hamsadanda—The traditional hamsadanda ("swan-staff"), or short crutch, is a T-frame typically made of wood or some other natural, energy-conducting material. It is placed in the armpit to apply pressure to the nerve plexus located there, which, when pressurized, can open the nostril on the opposite side of the body, thus affecting the corresponding current of bodily energy. Use of the hamsadanda in this manner can help balance the natural energies of the body.

Most Perfect / Most Ultimate—Avatar Adi Da uses the phrase "Most Perfect(ly)" in the sense of "Absolutely Perfect(ly)". Similarly, the phrase "Most Ultimate(ly)" is equivalent to "Absolutely Ultimate(ly)". "Most Perfect(ly)" and "Most Ultimate(ly)" are always references to the seventh (or Divinely Enlightened) stage of life. Avatar Adi Da uses "Perfect(ly)" and "Ultimate(ly)" (without "Most") to refer to the practice and realization in the context of the "Perfect Practice" of the Reality-Way of Adidam (or, when making reference to other traditions, to practice and realization in the context of the sixth stage of life).

"own-body Yogic sexual practice"—Avatar Adi Da describes sexual activity as a matter of individual, and (specifically) "own-body", responsibility. The "own-body Yogic sexual practice" is a means for an individual to learn about, and (thereafter) to rightly manage, sexual energy in his or her own body, in the context of the practice of devotion to Avatar Adi Da. The "own-body Yogic sexual practice" is (potentially) engaged by all Congregationist practitioners of Adidam, regardless of whether they are (in their personal intimate contexts) sexually active or celibate.

The "own-body Yogic sexual practice" involves Yogic self-stimulation, with the intention to "conduct" the natural energy in the circular energy pathway of the body-mind (while entirely avoiding degenerative orgasm). For devotees of Avatar Adi Da who have been Transcendentally Spiritually Initiated by Him, "own-body Yogic sexual practice" involves the "conductivity" of Avatar Adi Da's Transcendental Spiritual Energy in the natural circular pathway of the body-mind.

"Polarity screens"—Also called "Eeman screens" (after their inventor, L. E. Eeman), polarity screens consist of two screens of copper mesh to which wires with copper handles are attached. One screen is placed under the supine body at the lower spine and the other at the base of the head. One handle is held in each hand while the individual relaxes for ten to fifteen minutes on the screens to allow the realignment and energization of the etheric circuitry (or natural field of energy) of the body. ("Polarity plates", made of solid copper plates, may be used in the same fashion.) See *Polarity Screens: A Safe, Simple, and Naturally Effective Method for Restoring and Balancing the Energies of the Body, Based on the Practical Instruction of Adi Da (The Da Avatar)* for a more detailed explanation.

pranayama—Sanskrit for "restraint or regulation (yama) of life-energy (prana)". Pranayama is a technique for balancing, purifying, and intensifying the entire psycho-physical system by controlling the currents of the breath and life-force.

"radical"—Derived from the Latin "radix" (meaning "root"), "radical" principally means "irreducible", "fundamental", or "relating to the origin". Thus, Avatar Adi Da defines "radical" as "at-the-root". Because Avatar Adi Da uses "radical" in this literal sense, it appears in quotation marks in His writings, in order to distinguish His usage from the common reference to an extreme (often political) view.

"radical" devotion, right life, and "Perfect Knowledge"—The three fundamentals of the Reality-Way of Adidam. The practice of devotional turning to Avatar Adi Da—which He calls "radical" devotion because it occurs "at the root", prior to the body-mind—is based on devotional recognition and response to Avatar Adi Da as the Avatar, the incarnation of Reality. Once that basic foundation is established and demonstrated by right life (or steady embrace of the functional, practical, relational and cultural disciplines given by Avatar Adi Da), devotees are initiated into the technical form of practice Avatar Adi Da calls "the preliminary practice of 'Perfect Knowledge'". "Perfect Knowledge" is the tacit realization of Reality that is Avatar Adi Da's constant gift. Such "Knowledge" is, as Avatar Adi Da says, not of the mind—rather, "Perfect Knowledge" is "Reality Itself, As Is".

right life / right-life obedience—see **"radical" devotion, right life, and "Perfect Knowledge"**.

stages of life—Avatar Adi Da Samraj has "mapped" the potential developmental course of human experience as it unfolds through the gross, subtle, and causal dimensions of the being, describing this course in terms of six stages of life. These six stages of life, He explains, account for, and correspond with, all possible orientations to religion and culture that have arisen in human history. His own Divine Avataric Revelation—the Realization of the "Bright", or Reality Itself, Prior to all experience—He describes as the seventh stage of life.

The first three (or foundation) stages of life constitute the ordinary course of human adaptation—bodily, emotional, and mental growth. Each of the first three stages of life takes approximately seven years to be established. Every individual who lives to an adult age inevitably adapts (although, generally speaking, only partially) to the first three stages of life. In the general case, this is where the developmental process stops— at the gross level of adaptation. Traditions based fundamentally on beliefs and moral codes (without direct experience of the dimensions beyond the material world) belong to this foundation level of human development.

The fourth stage of life is characterized, in its beginnings, by a deep impulse to Communion with the Divine, felt to be a great "Other" in Whom the being aspires to become absorbed through devotional love and service. In the fifth stage of life, attention naturally moves into the domain of subtle experience and seeks the Samadhi states associated with ascending energy in the spinal line. The esoteric Spiritual traditions associated with mystical experience correspond with this higher level of human potential.

The Realizer of the sixth stage of life is focused in the causal depth of the being. He or she identifies with Consciousness (in profound states of meditation) by excluding all awareness of phenomena, both gross and subtle. And, when phenomena do arise, the sixth stage Realizer stands as the "Witness" of phenomena, unimplicated by body, mind, or world. Such is genuine Realization of the sixth stage of life—but Avatar Adi Da has also pointed out the tendency in some traditional circles to attempt to identify with Consciousness (or "the Self") based on a "talking"-school approach that is founded in mind, rather than genuine Realization.

The seventh stage of life, or the Realization of the "Bright" Reality Revealed through the Incarnation of Avatar Adi Da Samraj, transcends this entire six-stage course of human potential. In that Awakening, it is suddenly, tacitly Realized that there is no "difference" between Consciousness Itself and the "objects" of Consciousness. Thus, the seventh stage Realization wipes away every trace of dissociation from the body-mind and the world. Consciousness Itself, or Being Itself, Is all there is, and Consciousness Itself is found to be Radiant, or Love-Bliss-Full. Thus, every "thing" and every "one" that appears is inherently recognized to be a mere modification of the One Divine "Brightness" (or the Divine Conscious Light).

student-beginner—The student-beginner phase of practice is the first phase of practice in the First Congregation of Adidam. Before entering the First Congregation as a student-beginner, the devotee practices within the Second Congregation, establishing the foundation practice of "radical" devotion to Avatar Adi Da and adapting to the right-life-disciplines of the Reality-Way of Adidam. Once that initial foundation has been established, the individual is acknowledged to be prepared for entrance into the First Congregation, and is thereupon initiated into the preliminary listening-practice of "Perfect Knowledge" as a student-beginner. See also **"radical" devotion, right life, and "Perfect Knowledge"**.

Transcendental Spiritual—A principal description used by Avatar Adi Da Samraj of the unique nature of the process in His Company. "Transcendental" refers to the Consciousness aspect of Reality, and "Spiritual" refers to the Energy aspect of Reality—thus, with the phrase "Transcendental Spiritual" Avatar Adi Da communicates the inherent Coincidence of the two (ultimate and co-equal) aspects of Reality that is His Realization and Revelation: the One and Only and Inherently Indivisible Conscious Light Itself. This coincidence sets Avatar Adi Da's Revelation and Way apart from all traditional forms of Realization. The esoteric traditions of Transcendental Realization (or Realization of Consciousness) involve dissociative introversion, whereby the body and the world are excluded—thereby excluding the Energy (or Spiritual) dimension of Reality. Likewise, all traditional forms of Spirituality are practiced on the "platform" of identification with the body-mind-"self", and not from the prior disposition of identification with Consciousness Itself—thereby subordinating or dissociated from the Consciousness (or Transcendental) aspect of Existence. In contrast, the Transcendental Spirituality of Adidam is the Spiritual (or Energy) process that is founded in the transcending of identification with the body-mind-"self"—without any act of dissociation from anything whatsoever. Thus, the Reality-Way Revealed by Avatar Adi Da Samraj is unique among all traditions of esoteric Realization.

Yogic "conductivity" massage—A specific form of massage, Given by Avatar Adi Da, that enhances the flow of life-energy (and, as the case may be, Avatar Adi Da's Transcendental Spiritual Energy) in the body-mind, by massaging in the pattern of the circuit of the body-mind—up the back and down the front.

APPENDIX A

Online Reference Charts

The following URLs link to standard reference charts for height, weight, caloric intake, body mass index, and so forth. While these can be useful in monitoring one's adaptation to and maintenance of the raw diet, keep in mind that all such standardized charts are made on the basis of conventional dietary practices, not the searchless raw dietary approach.

Height/Weight Chart:

http://www.healthchecksystems.com/heightweightchart.htm

Calorie Intake Recommendations:

http://www.dinewise.com/calorie_calculator

Calories in Specific Foods:

http://www.thecaloriecounter.com/

Body Mass Index Charts / Calculators:

http://www.consumer.gov/weightloss/bmi.htm

http://www.cdc.gov/nccdphp/dnpa/bmi/

Glycemic Index and Load:

http://www.mendosa.com/gilists.htm

Or see the "Database" search function on this site:

http://www.glycemicindex.com/

Food Database and Other Reference Charts:

(search specific foods for nutritional info)

www.nutritiondata.com

Food Combining Information:

http://www.rawfoodchat.com/forums/raw-food-lifestyle-
lounge/fruit-question-1227.html

See also *Food Combining Made Easy* by Herbert M. Shelton.
(San Antonio, TX: Willow Publishing, 1940).
ISBN 0-9606948-0-3.

Or you can buy the below guide for US$6.00:

http://foodnsport.com/max2/catalog/product_info.php?
products_id=106&osCsid=3b83ecf29a8b6e4cce5058b3791ed85e

APPENDIX B

How to Do an Enema

1. Use a collapsible rubber 1-quart (or 1-liter) enema bag. Rinse bag, nozzle, and tube.

2. Fill the enema bag with enema liquid (generally tepid water). Mildly warm water is the least shocking to the bowel mucosa and muscles. Use pure, unchlorinated water.

3. Connect enema bag with enema tube, and enema tube with enema nozzle.

4. Clamp enema tube.

5. Hang the enema bag at a height of about five feet. (Adjust to a lower height if it causes too much pressure.)

6. Assume the all-fours position (on your knees and elbows), on the floor.

7. Lubricate your anus and the nozzle with a natural oil or lubricant.

8. Insert the nozzle into your anus.

9. Release the clamp and let the enema liquid flow into the colon. Remember to breathe deeply and relax bodily.

10. Clamp the tubing as soon as there is a sensation of "fullness" or when the enema bag is empty.

11. From the all-fours position, or bending your elbows and placing the head on your hands, begin some light stomach rolls (for Avatar Adi Da's recommended form of stomach rolls, please see *Conscious Exercise and The Transcendental Sun* or the *Conscious Exercise* video available through the Dawn Horse Press). You may also massage the abdomen—starting from the left lower quadrant up to and under the left lower ribcage area, then across to under the right side, and then down to the right

lower quadrant. Both the exercising and massage move the water beyond the sigmoid colon (on the left side), up the descending colon and along the transverse colon, and even over to the right side down to the junction of the colon with the small intestine. The further the water goes around, the better the cleanse.

12. If you can (and if some water remains in the enema bag), allow more or all of the remaining water to flow into the rectum/colon.

13. When all the water has run in or you have reached your limit, re-clamp the enema tube and then remove the nozzle from your anus.

14. Now stand up and do more stomach rolls and massage as described previously, as well as exercises such as windmill, waist bends, and walking in place, as indicated by Avatar Adi Da in *Conscious Exercise and The Transcendental Sun.* Note: Do the exercises lightly and slowly, with the purpose of moving the water to the right lower part of the colon.

15. Preferably, and without forcing yourself, retain the enema for five to twenty minutes.

16. Empty your bowel completely.

17. After emptying your bowel, you can repeat the process, although over time when you become experienced with this procedure, once is generally enough.

18. If you cannot hold a full quart (or liter) of enema liquid, take several smaller enemas until you learn to absorb the full amount into the bowel and are able to hold it there for fifteen to thirty minutes.

19. For your first enemas during a fast, you may want to repeat the procedure several times, until the colon is totally clean (that is, until the return water is clear and not discolored). The best results are achieved by massaging the intestines and by holding the water as long as possible/comfortable.

The Liver Flush

The liver flush optimally requires three to six days of preparation—eating raw or (if you have not yet adapted to the totally raw diet) nearly raw (as you would do in preparing for a fast), with the last day being sixteen to twenty hours of actual cleansing (eating only raw, cleansing fruits and/or vegetables). Please consult a licensed health practitioner before engaging this process.

You will need the following items:

- Oral Epsom salts: 4 tablespoons/60g (to be dissolved in 24 oz. [3 cups/700 ml] of water)

- Virgin olive oil, cold pressed: 4 oz. (½ cup/120 ml)

- Either fresh grapefruit or fresh lemon, or fresh lemon and orange combined

Best time for the liver flush:

Plan your preparation (eating raw) such that the flush itself is on the weekend (or other days when you are not required to go to work).

Make sure that you do an enema before and after the flush.

The day of the flush:

- If you feel hungry in the morning, eat a light breakfast.

- Do not eat any protein foods or fats in any form.

- Do not eat or drink anything (except water) after 1:30 p.m.

The Actual Cleanse:

Evening

6:00 p.m.: Add four tablespoons (60g) of <u>oral</u> Epsom salts (magnesium sulfate) to 24 oz. (3 cups/700 ml) of filtered (or distilled) water in a jar. This makes four servings, 6 oz. (¾ cup/175 ml) each. Drink your first serving at 6 p.m. You may take a few sips of water afterward to get rid of the bitter taste in the mouth or add a little lemon juice to the dissolved Epsom salts to improve the taste. Some people drink it with a large plastic straw to bypass the taste buds on the tongue. You may want to brush your teeth afterward or rinse out the mouth with baking soda. If thirsty, you may drink some water before the second serving of Epsom salts. (If you are allergic to Epsom salts or are just not able to get it down, you may instead use the second best choice—magnesium citrate—at the same dosage.)

8:00 p.m.: Drink your second serving of 6 oz. (¾ cup/175 ml) of Epsom salts in water.

9:30 p.m.: If you have not had a bowel movement until now and have not done a colon cleanse within twenty-four hours, take a water enema. This will trigger a series of bowel movements.

9:45 p.m.: Squeeze the grapefruit (or lemons, or lemons and oranges) and strain the pulp from the juice. You will need 6 oz. (¾ cup/175 ml) of juice. Pour the juice and 4 oz. (½ cup/120 ml) of olive oil into 16 oz. (2 cups/500ml) jar. Close the jar tightly and shake hard, about twenty times or until the solution is watery.

10:00 p.m.: Stand next to your bed (do not sit down) and drink the mixture of juice and olive oil, if possible, straight. Some people prefer to drink it through a large plastic straw. Most people have no problem drinking it straight, but, if necessary, take a little honey between sips, which helps the mixture to be more palatable. Do not take more than five minutes to complete drinking the mixture.

Lie down, with lights out, on your back, with one or two pillows propping you up so that your head is higher than your abdomen. If this is uncomfortable, lie on your right side, with your knees pulled towards your head. Lie perfectly still for at least twenty minutes. Go to sleep if you can. If you cannot fall asleep, remain in bed nevertheless.

Only get up if you feel the urge to have a bowel movement. Check for stones every time you go to the bathroom. You may feel nauseated during the night and/or in the early morning hours. The nausea will pass as the morning progresses.

The Following Morning

6:00–6:30 a.m.: Upon awakening, but not before 6 a.m., drink your third 6 oz. (¾ cup/175 ml) of Epsom salts (if you feel very thirsty drink a glass of water before taking the salts). Rest, read, or meditate. If you are very sleepy, you may go back to bed, although it is best if the body stays in an upright position. Most people feel absolutely fine and prefer to do some light stretching exercises, such as Hatha Yoga. Do not take any food at this time.

8:00–8:30 a.m.: Drink your fourth and last 6 oz. (¾ cup/175 ml) of Epsom salts.

10:00–10:30 a.m.: You may drink freshly pressed fruit juice at this time. Thirty minutes later you may eat one or two pieces of fresh fruit.

Do an enema thirty minutes later.

One hour after the enema, you may eat a light meal of solid food. By the evening or the next morning, your digestive system should be back to normal and you should feel the first signs of improvement.

Drink adequate water.

Continue to eat light meals during the following days.

Do daily enemas for two to three days, as needed.

APPENDIX D

De La Torre's Drink

The recipe for the basic "de la Torre" drink is as follows:

Wash but do not peel the following vegetables and cut them into small cubes. Put them into a jar with 48 oz. (6 cups [1.5 liters]) of spring water, if possible, to leach out the water-soluble vitamins and minerals.

> 6 oz. [180 ml] carrots
>
> 4 oz. [120 ml] beets
>
> 2 oz. [60 ml] celery
>
> 2 leaves peppermint

Let the vegetables soak three to six hours or overnight in the refrigerator, stirring once or twice. Strain out 8 oz. (1 cup [240 ml]) at a time, as needed, leaving the vegetables in the jar. When there are one or two glasses of liquid left, add one more glass of water to dilute it. [From *The Process of Physical Purification by Means of the New and Easy Way to Fast: An Extraordinary, Transcendental Discovery in Body Purification, Showing an Easy and Fast Way to a Higher Degree of Health and Longer Span of Life*, by Teofilo de la Torre (Costa Rica: 1957), pp. 74–78.]

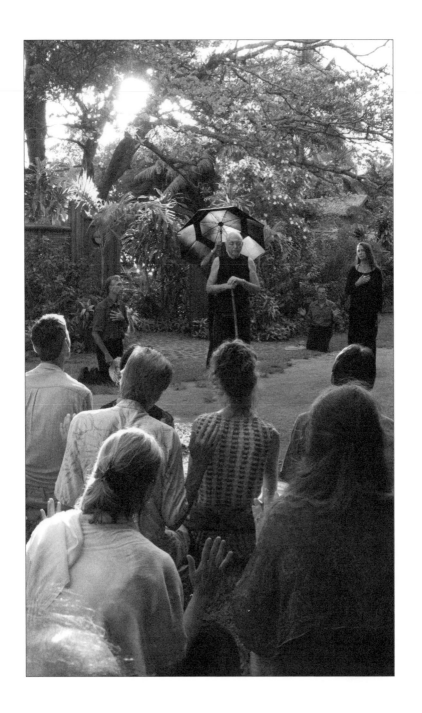

Become a Formal Devotee of His Divine Presence The Divine Avataric World-Teacher Ruchira Avatar Adi Da Samraj

Adidam is not a conventional "religion".
Adidam is not a conventional way of life.
Adidam is about the transcending of the ego-"I".
Adidam is about the Freedom of Divine Self-Realization.

Adidam is not based on mythology or belief.
Adidam is a Reality-practice.
Adidam is a "reality consideration", in which the various modes of egoity are directly transcended.

Adidam is a universally applicable Way of life.
Adidam is for those who will choose It, and whose hearts and intelligence fully respond to Me and My Offering.
Adidam is a Great Revelation, and It is to be freely and openly communicated to all.

—His Divine Presence
Ruchira Avatar Adi Da Samraj

In the depth of every being lies the inherent heart-impulse to be completely and utterly Free. In this book, you have been introduced to the Reality-Revelation of His Divine Presence Ruchira Avatar Adi Da Samraj, Who not only Speaks directly to this impulse, but Who <u>Is</u> That Freedom, Communicating Itself directly to you, and to all beings.

Ruchira Avatar Adi Da's Birth in 1939 was an intentional embrace of the human situation, for the sake of Revealing the Way of Divine Liberation to all and Offering the

Transcendental Spiritual Blessing that Awakens the Realization of Prior Freedom. His Divine Presence Adi Da Samraj is thus the fulfillment of the ancient intuitions of the "Avatar"—the One Who Appears in human Form, as a direct manifestation of Reality Itself.

In an unprecedented Teaching-Revelation process (beginning in 1972, and now complete), Ruchira Avatar Adi Da Samraj spoke for countless hours with those who recognized and devotionally responded to Him—always looking for them, as representatives of humanity, to ask all of their questions about God, Truth, Reality, and human life. In response, Avatar Adi Da Samraj created a vast body of Written and Spoken Teaching in which He Communicates in every detail the means for, and the signs of, ecstatic ego-transcending participation in the Direct Revelation of Reality Itself—As It Is, prior to body and mind and self and world. Thus, Avatar Adi Da created a new tradition based on His direct Avataric Revelation of Reality Itself: the "Radical" Reality-Way of Adidam Ruchiradam, which is the devotional and Transcendental Spiritual relationship to Avatar Adi Da Samraj.

Ruchira Avatar Adi Da's True Function as Spiritual Master is not to teach or somehow magically "cause" Realization in His devotees. Rather, Avatar Adi Da's Function is to simply Be—As He Is, As the Divine Reality-State—and thus to make available to all beings the Direct Revelation of Reality Itself and the Means to Realize It. If you are moved to take up His Way, Avatar Adi Da Samraj invites you to enter into a direct and real devotional and Transcendental Spiritual relationship to Him.

To find His Divine Presence Ruchira Avatar Adi Da Samraj is to find the Very Heart of Reality—tangibly "known", prior to body and mind, as the Deepest Truth of Existence. This is the great mystery you are invited to discover. ■

I am not simply *Speaking* to those who are already *My* formal devotees. *I am Speaking to everyone—literally.*

I Meditate everybody. I Am everybody. And I am Speaking to everybody—but not to everybody as egos. I am Speaking to "everybody-all-at-once"—at the Heart, at the Place Where I Am. In that Place, there are no "differences". Where there are no "differences", people come to Me and are able to "Locate" Me and Commune with Me.

Adidam is not about egos. Adidam is not about an identity that comes through "belonging". Adidam is participation in the Divine.

You can participate in the Divine only in the Place of the Divine. The Divine Is a Place intrinsically without ego. The Divine is not a place you are "moving to". The Divine Is the Place Where you Are—Always Already.

The Divine Is Where there is no ego and no "other". Where there is an "other", there is no Real God, no Truth. Reality Itself Is Where there is no "other".

The Only Room That Is Is the Room in Which there is no "other", no "point of view"—but Only Real God, Only That Which Is Divine, Self-Existing, Self-Radiant, Indivisible, Acausal, Intrinsically egoless, Outshining all-and-All.

That is the "Temple" of Adidam. And That Is Where everybody Is—Always Already and egolessly.

—His Divine Presence
Ruchira Avatar Adi Da Samraj
May 31, 2008

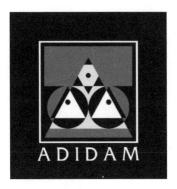

On the following pages are a number of ways that you can choose to deepen your response to Avatar Adi Da and to consider becoming His formal devotee.

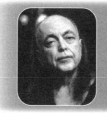

**Visit the
Adidam website:
www.adidam.org**

- **SEE AUDIO-VISUAL PRESENTATIONS** on the Divine Life and Transcendental Spiritual Revelation of Avatar Adi Da Samraj

- **LISTEN TO DISCOURSES** Given by Avatar Adi Da
  - Transcending egoic notions of God
  - Why Reality cannot be grasped by the mind
  - How the devotional relationship to Avatar Adi Da moves you beyond ego-bondage
  - The supreme process of Spiritual Transmission

- **READ QUOTATIONS** from the "Source-Texts" of Avatar Adi Da Samraj
  - Real (Acausal) God as the <u>only</u> Reality
  - The ancient practice of devotion to the Realizer
  - The two opposing life-strategies characteristic of the West and the East—and the way beyond both
  - The Prior Unity at the root of all that exists
  - The limits of scientific materialism
  - The true Way beyond all seeking
  - The esoteric structure of the human being
  - The real process of death and reincarnation
  - The nature of Divine Enlightenment

- **SUBSCRIBE** to the online *Adidam Revelation* magazine

THE AVATAR OF WHAT IS

The Divine Life and Work of Adi Da

by Carolyn Lee, PhD

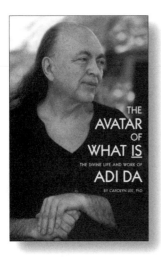

This new biography presents a summary overview of Avatar Adi Da's Life and Work from His Birth to the present time. From the foretelling of His Birth, through His years of "Learning humankind", to the more than thirty-five years of His unique Avataric Teaching-and-Blessing-Work, this is the extraordinary story of Avatar Adi Da's Divine Intervention in the world.

The Purpose of My bodily (human) Appearance here is the Divine Liberation of all of humankind—not merely the human beings of the East or the human beings of the West, but all human beings (and, indeed, all beings and things altogether).

—His Divine Presence Ruchira Avatar Adi Da Samraj

Avatar Adi Da's Divine Emergence marks a new chapter in epochal Spiritual History.

—RICHARD GROSSINGER
Author, *Planet Medicine, The Night Sky,* and *Embryogenesis*

The life and teaching of Avatar Adi Da are of profound and decisive spiritual significance at this critical moment in history.

—BRYAN DESCHAMP
Senior Adviser at the United Nations
High Commission for Refugees

There exists nowhere in the world today, among Christians, Jews, Muslims, Hindus, Buddhists, native tribalists, or any other groups, anyone who has so much to teach, or speaks with such authority, or is so important for understanding our situation. If we are willing to learn from him in every way, he is a Pole around which the world can get its bearings.

—HENRY LEROY FINCH
Author, *Wittgenstein—The Early Philosophy*
and *Wittgenstein—The Later Philosophy*

152 pp., **$12.95**

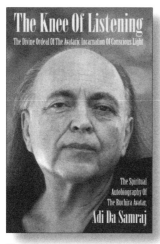

THE KNEE OF LISTENING

The Divine Ordeal Of
The Avataric Incarnation
Of Conscious Light

The Spiritual Autobiography
of His Divine Presence
Ruchira Avatar Adi Da Samraj

Born in 1939 on Long Island, New York, Avatar Adi Da Samraj describes His earliest Life as an existence of constant and unmitigated Spiritual "Brightness". His observation, still in infancy, that others did not live in this manner led Him to undertake an awesome quest—to discover why human beings suffer and how they can transcend that suffering. His quest led Him to a confrontation with the bleak despair of post-industrial Godlessness, to a minute examination of the workings of subjective awareness, to discipleship in a lineage of profound Yogis, to a period of intense Christian mysticism, and finally to a Re-Awakening to the perfect state of "Brightness" He had known at Birth.

In *The Knee of Listening*, Avatar Adi Da also reveals His own direct awareness of His "deeper-personality vehicles"—the beings whose lives were the direct antecedents (or the "pre-history") of His present human Lifetime—the great nineteenth-century Indian Realizers Sri Ramakrishna and Swami Vivekananda. Finally, Avatar Adi Da describes the series of profound transformational events that took place in the decades after His Divine Re-Awakening—each one a form of "Yogic death" for which there is no recorded precedent.

Altogether, *The Knee of Listening* is the unparalleled history of how the Divine Conscious Light has Incarnated in human form, in order to grant everyone the possibility of Ultimate Divine Liberation, Freedom, and Happiness.

The Knee of Listening *is without a doubt the most profound Spiritual autobiography of all time.*

—ROGER SAVOIE, PhD
Philosopher; translator; author, *La Vipère et le Lion:*
La Voie radicale de la Spiritualité

822 pp., **$24.95**

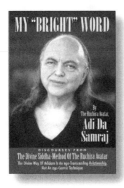

MY "BRIGHT" WORD

by His Divine Presence
Ruchira Avatar Adi Da Samraj

New edition of the classic Spiritual
Discourses originally published as
The Method of the Siddhas

In these Talks from the early years of His
Teaching-Work, Avatar Adi Da gives extraordinary
Instruction on the foundation of True Spiritual life,
covering topics such as the primary mechanism
by which we are preventing the Realization of
Truth, the means to overcome this mechanism, and the true function of the
Spiritual Master in relation to the devotee.

In modern language, this volume teaches the ancient all-time
trans-egoic truths. It transforms the student by paradox and by example.
Consciousness, understanding, and finally the awakened Self are the
rewards. What more can anyone want? **—ELMER GREEN, PhD**
Director Emeritus, Center for Applied Psychophysiology,
The Menninger Clinic

544 pp., **$24.95**

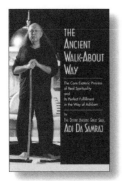

THE ANCIENT WALK-ABOUT WAY

The Core Esoteric Process of Real Spirituality
and Its Perfect Fulfillment in
the Way of Adidam

In this beautiful collection of essays, His Divine
Presence Ruchira Avatar Adi Da begins with a
foundation consideration of the purpose and principles of the ancient tradition of heart-response to
the living Realizer; He then describes how to culti-
vate life-conditions that allow the being to enact
its inherent heart-response to Living Truth; and,
finally, He describes the unique Signs and Qualities of His Appearance
and Offering, and of those who fully devotionally respond to Him.

Devotion to the Realizer is the ancient Way of true Spiritual life.
Devotion to the Realizer is the "pre-civilization Way", which existed before
any recorded history, during a time when human beings were, essentially,
merely wandering all over the Earth. Devotion to the Realizer has always
been the fundamental Means of human Spirituality.
—His Divine Presence Ruchira Avatar Adi Da Samraj

144 pp., **$12.95**

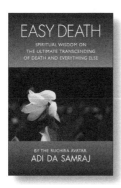

EASY DEATH

Spiritual Wisdom on the Ultimate
Transcending of Death and Everything Else
by His Divine Presence
Ruchira Avatar Adi Da Samraj

This 2005 edition of *Easy Death* is thoroughly revised and updated with:

■ Talks and essays from Avatar Adi Da on death and ultimate transcendence

■ Accounts of profound events of Yogic death in Avatar Adi Da's own Life

■ Stories of His Blessing in the death transitions of His devotees

. . . an exciting, stimulating, and thought-provoking book that adds immensely to the ever-increasing literature on the phenomena of life and death. But, more important, perhaps, it is a confirmation that a life filled with love instead of fear can lead to ultimately meaningful life and death. Thank you for this masterpiece.

—ELISABETH KÜBLER-ROSS, MD
Author, *On Death and Dying*

544 pp., **$24.95**

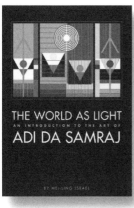

THE WORLD AS LIGHT

An Introduction to the Art
of Adi Da Samraj
by Mei-Ling Israel

The condition of non-separateness—as the true nature of the human situation, and the true nature of Reality altogether—is the core of Avatar Adi Da's communication in His art. This generously illustrated book provides an overview of the massive body of highly distinctive artwork Avatar Adi Da Samraj has created over the past forty years—accompanied by key statements He has made on His own art and on the artistic process in general. Published on the occasion of Avatar Adi Da's collateral exhibition at the 52nd Biennale di Venezia (2007).

The living body always wants (with wanting need) to allow the Light of Perfect Reality into the "room". Assisting human beings to fulfill that impulse is what I work to do by every act of image-art.
—His Divine Presence Ruchira Avatar Adi Da Samraj

128 pp., with over 140 color and black-and-white illustrations, **$24.95**

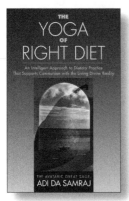

THE YOGA OF RIGHT DIET

*An Intelligent Approach to Dietary Practice That
Supports Communion with the Living Divine Reality*
by His Divine Presence
Ruchira Avatar Adi Da Samraj

*The practice of diet is simply an ordinary discipline for
intelligent people who are devoted to always present
Communion with the Living Divine Reality, Truth, and
Real (Acausal) God.*

—His Divine Presence Ruchira Avatar Adi Da Samraj

What you will find in this book is not the usual information regarding health,
but rather a unique description of diet and healing from a "point of view" that is
entirely "radical".

Avatar Adi Da's approach to the matter of diet and health is both straightforward and profound. He says that true "food" is Reality Itself, and that true health
is "about sustenance, about love, and not really about conventional matters of diet
and health". Thus, to truly be healthy, one must locate the True Source-Condition
of all that appears, and it is from there that healing can occur.

—from the introduction by Charles Seage, MD
88 pp., **$12.95**

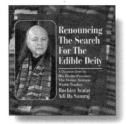

RENOUNCING THE SEARCH
FOR THE EDIBLE DEITY

In this remarkable Talk, Avatar Adi Da Samraj describes
how the shock of (apparently) independent existence initi-
ates the false search for the "edible deity"—or the "food"
that is perfectly sustaining. What is truly required, He says,
is not any outside source of sustenance, but to transcend
the contraction upon "self" by entering into Divine Communion—to the point of
discovering Perfect Sustenance, our True Condition of Perfect Non-separateness
from Reality.

*If you could simply feel your Condition, feel as your Condition in this moment,
without obstruction, without making an interpretation, then you would not be in
the condition of obstructed feeling-attention, in that case, defining yourself, feeling
vulnerable, separate, a being. And you would discover, directly, intuitively, the Nature
of your Condition—Which in no sense is separated out, Which Is Pure, Absolute
Energy without qualification, Which is sustained Absolutely, Which was never
separated from anything, Which does not exist in an inherently separated state.*

—His Divine Presence Ruchira Avatar Adi Da Samraj
CD, running time: 52 minutes
$16.95

THE ADIDAM REVELATION DISCOURSES
on DVD

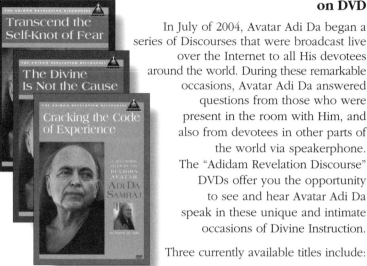

In July of 2004, Avatar Adi Da began a series of Discourses that were broadcast live over the Internet to all His devotees around the world. During these remarkable occasions, Avatar Adi Da answered questions from those who were present in the room with Him, and also from devotees in other parts of the world via speakerphone. The "Adidam Revelation Discourse" DVDs offer you the opportunity to see and hear Avatar Adi Da speak in these unique and intimate occasions of Divine Instruction.

Three currently available titles include:

TRANSCEND THE SELF-KNOT OF FEAR
Running time: 60 minutes. Includes subtitles in English, Spanish, French, German, Dutch, and Polish.

THE DIVINE IS NOT THE CAUSE
Running time: 72 minutes. Includes subtitles in English, Spanish, French, German, Dutch, Finnish, Polish, Czech, Chinese, Japanese, and Hebrew.

CRACKING THE CODE OF EXPERIENCE
Running time: 86 minutes. Includes subtitles in English, Spanish, German, Dutch, Polish, Czech, Chinese, Japanese, and Hebrew.

DVD, **$26.95** each

THE DAWN HORSE PRESS

1-877-770-0772
(from within North America)

1-707-928-6653
(from outside North America)

www.dawnhorsepress.com

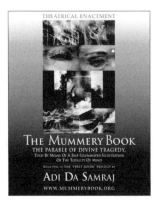
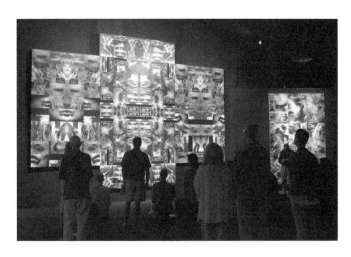

Support Avatar Adi Da's Work
and the Reality-Way of Adidam

■ If you are moved to serve Avatar Adi Da's Work specifically through advocacy and/or financial patronage, please contact:

Advocacy
12180 Ridge Road
Middletown, CA 95461
phone: (707) 928-5267
email: adidam_advocacy@adidam.org

For young people:
Join the Adidam Youth Fellowship

■ Young people under 21 can participate in the "Adidam Youth Fellowship"—either as a "friend" or practicing member. Adidam Youth Fellowship members participate in study programs, retreats, celebrations, and other events with other young people responding to Avatar Adi Da. To learn more about the Youth Fellowship, call or write:

Vision of Mulund Institute (VMI)
10336 Loch Lomond Road, PMB 146
Middletown, CA 95461
phone: (707) 928-6932
email: vmi@adidam.org
www.visionofmulund.org

Fear-No-More Zoo and Gardens

■ To learn more about Avatar Adi Da's regard for non-humans, visit:
www.fearnomorezoo.org
Or call or write:
Fear-No-More Zoo and Gardens
12040 North Seigler Road
Middletown, CA 95461, USA
phone: (707) 355-0638

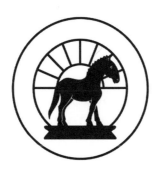

To order books, tapes, CDs, DVDs,
and videos by and about
His Divine Presence Ruchira Avatar Adi Da Samraj,
contact

THE DAWN HORSE PRESS

1-877-770-0772
(from within North America)

1-707-928-6653
(from outside North America)

Or visit the Dawn Horse Press website:

www.dawnhorsepress.com

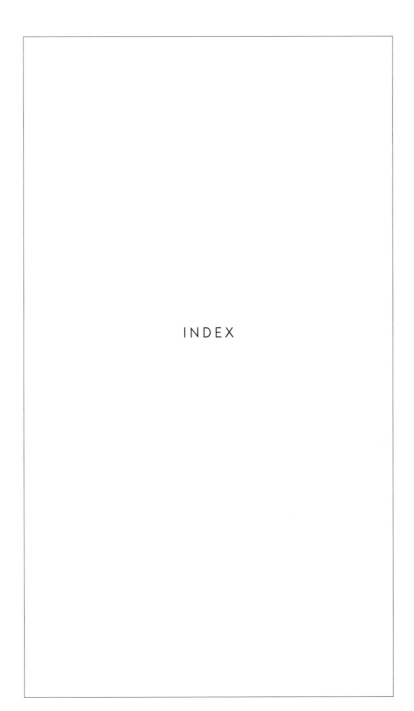

INDEX

A

adaptation process. *See* dietary transitions
addicts, human beings as, 68
Adi Da Samraj
books on diet by, 9, 34n, 66, 87
devotional relationship to, 12, 16
Life and offering of, 15–16
Reality-Teaching of, 15, 45–47, 72–73
Teaching-Submission of, 11, 43–44, 72–73
Adi Da Samrajashram, 9
Adidam.org website, 165
Adidam Ruchiradam, 143
Avatar Adi Da's Revelation of, 15–16
congregations of, 144
culture of good company in, 76–77
devotional basis for, 22, 83
dietary discipline in, 12, 25–26, 55, 73, 78–79
right-life practice in, 21, 55, 60–61, 80–81, 83
three fundamentals of, 147
alcohol, 39, 41
Aletheon, The (Adi Da Samraj), 15, 139
algae, 30, 106, 115
alkaloids, 69, 115
allopathy, 78
aluminum utensils, 112
animal products, 38, 97
animals
ancient sacrifice of, 70
industrial killing of, 70–72
autonomic nervous system, 90–91

B

bad company, 76
balancing phase of healing, 90–91, 93
Basket of Tolerance, The (Adi Da Samraj), 131
black tea, 28, 107
blender drinks. *See* green drinks
blenders, 65, 114
blue-green algae, 30, 106, 115
body-mind-complex
dimensions of, 24
effect of food-taking on, 22–23
preventing illness in, 60
re-sensitization to, 57
Bouwmeester, Daniel, 12
bowel functioning, 123
BPA (Bisphenol-A), 112
"Bright", the, 143

C

caffeine, 28, 107
causal dimension, 24
change, secret of, 139–41
charts, reference, 151–52
children, fasting by, 127
chlorella, 30, 63, 106, 115
chocolate, 106
citrus fruits, 129
coffee, 28, 107
"conductivity" practice, 25, 112, 143
congregations of Adidam, 144
"conscious exercise", 100, 112, 144
Conscious Exercise and The Transcendental Sun (Adi Da Samraj), 87, 153, 154
conservative diet, 26

ADIDAM

Find out more about His Divine Presence *Ruchira Avatar Adi Da Samraj* and the Reality-Way of Adidam

■ Find out about courses, seminars, events, and retreats by calling the regional center nearest you.

AMERICAS
12040 N. Seigler Rd.
Middletown, CA
95461 USA
1-707-928-4936

THE UNITED KINGDOM
uk@adidam.org
0845-330-1008

EUROPE-AFRICA
Annendaalderweg 10
6105 AT Maria Hoop
The Netherlands
31 (0)20 468 1442

PACIFIC-ASIA
12 Seibel Road
Henderson
Auckland 0614
New Zealand
64-9-838-9114

AUSTRALIA
P.O. Box 244
Kew 3101
Victoria
**1800 ADIDAM
(1800-234-326)**

INDIA
F-168 Shree Love-Ananda Marg
Rampath, Shyam Nagar Extn.
Jaipur - 302 019, India
91 (141) 2293080

EMAIL: **correspondence@adidam.org**

■ Order books, tapes, CDs, DVDs, and videos by and about Ruchira Avatar Adi Da Samraj.
1-877-770-0772 (from within North America)
1-707-928-6653 (from outside North America)
order online: **www.dawnhorsepress.com**

■ Visit the Adidam website:
www.adidam.org
Discover more about Ruchira Avatar Adi Da Samraj and the Reality-Way of Adidam.